LIVING WITH MOTOR NEURONE DISEASE

A complete guide

Navigating the path following a life-changing diagnosis can be bewildering and exhausting. This wonderful book shines a guiding light on the road ahead with the help of experts who have walked it – the medics, the caregivers and, perhaps most importantly, those who are living with motor neurone disease. I know this guide will provide some comfort to those who are starting on this road and their families, whose burden will only be eased if we all commit to supporting them.

Claire Byrne, radio and TV presenter, RTÉ

Having travelled a little of the MND journey in the company of the wonderful Fr Tony Coote, I became aware of the complexity of this disease and its impact on patient, family, friends and carers. It would have been so helpful to Fr Tony and his support network to have had this *MindYourSelf* book *Living with Motor Neurone Disease: A complete guide*. I know that this book will be an essential resource for everyone who is affected in any way by the MND experience.

Professor Joe Carthy, college principal and dean of science, University College Dublin

Living with Motor Neurone Disease: A complete guide is a book that raises awareness and understanding of every aspect of living with MND. To those readers already fully aware, it offers compassionate and comprehensive guidance through the moments that lie ahead. This book would have been an invaluable help to myself and my brothers as we attempted to assist Tony through his illness. The IMNDA has been working on the front line in regard to patient care, well-being and rights since 1985. The IMNDA role is crucial in maintaining support for people diagnosed with this terrible illness until such time as the ongoing research develops a permanent cure. Funding is the cornerstone of all this good work, and supporting and contributing is now more important than ever. All royalties from this important book *Living with Motor Neurone Disease: A complete guide* will go directly to supporting the IMNDA.

Kieran Coote. Kieran is a brother of the late Fr Tony Coote who turned his diagnosis of MND into a mission to promote awareness of MND and to raise funds for Research Motor Neurone (www.rmn.ie) and the Irish Motor Neurone Disease Association (www.imnda.ie) through his 'Walk While You Can' campaign in which, over four weeks in 2018, he journeyed in a wheelchair from Donegal to Cork (www.wwyc.ie).

This new book in the Cork University Press *MindYourSelf* series, *Living with Motor Neurone Disease: A complete guide*, gives direction and hope to anyone affected by MND. It is beautifully detailed, technical, honest and authoritative on all aspects of MND. It is wonderful to see such a complete guide presented genuinely and sympathetically with the IMNDA motto that 'until there is a cure, there is care'. *Living with Motor Neurone Disease* is a publication that provides care through sensitive and informed direction, illustrating what care looks like from every aspect of need. I heartily recommend this book for anyone affected with, working in the area of, or wishing to learn more about this challenging condition. This book is a vital resource and also a gift full of insight and compassion.

Mary C. Morrissey, M.Sc., C.Psychol. FPsSI, psychology lead, Research and Evidence, HSE and principal clinical

psychologist, Connolly hospital; former president of the Psychological Society of Ireland

This is an important book. It is designed to be a complete guide to motor neurone disease and to provide all the information needed to negotiate a path through the challenges of this neurodegenerative condition. This book will be a useful, readable and knowledgeable resource for those diagnosed with motor neurone disease and their families. It also provides a guide for healthcare professionals involved in this specialist area.

Dr Bernadette Mangan, board director at St John of God hospital CLG; retired consultant psychiatrist and clinical director

Spending time with Fr Tony Coote after his diagnosis of motor neurone disease as his condition progressed rapidly and inexorably was a shocking wake-up to just how much there is to learn about MND, and how fast. This new book in the Cork University Press *MindYourSelf* series, *Living with Motor Neurone Disease: A complete guide*, is surely a vital accompaniment to anyone diagnosed, and their loved ones. It includes professional expertise, practical legal advice, information on how to talk to children and teenagers when a parent has a diagnosis, and far more. All delivered sympathetically with the IMNDA motto that 'until there is a cure, there is care'.

Emily Hourican, author

This book is dedicated to all those who are living with motor neurone disease, to their families who love and care for them, the multidisciplinary professionals who support them, to the researchers who seek new ways of understanding and ameliorating the impact of the diagnosis, and to all who so generously support the work of the Irish Motor Neurone Disease Association.

Those who have lost people they loved through MND are not forgotten. This dedication extends to everyone who has been bereaved by this condition.

Titles in the *MindYourSelf* Mental Health and Well-Being Series

Personal Struggles: Oppression, healing and liberation
Dr Sean Ruth
Published in 2019 ISBN 978-1-78205-348-4

Uncertainty Rules? Making uncertainty work for you
Richard Plenty and Terri Morrissey
Published in 2020 ISBN 978-1-78205-377-4

Rewriting Our Stories: Education, empowerment
and well-being
Dr Derek Gladwin
Published in 2021 ISBN 978-1-78205-417-7

LIVING WITH MOTOR NEURONE DISEASE

A complete guide

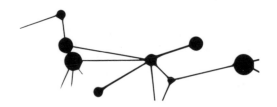

Edited by Dr Marie Murray

In collaboration with the Irish Motor Neurone
Disease Association

All contributor royalties go to the IMNDA

First published in 2021 by Atrium
Atrium is an imprint of Cork University Press
Boole Library
University College Cork
Cork T12 ND89
Ireland

Library of Congress Control Number: 2021936169

Distribution in the USA Longleaf Services, Chapel Hill,
NC, USA.

British Library Cataloguing in Publication Data
A CIP catalogue record for this book is available from the
British Library.

ISBN 9781782054832

Typeset by Studio 10 Design
Printed by Gutenberg Press in Malta

www.corkuniversitypress.com

DR MARIE MURRAY has worked as a clinical psychologist for more than forty years across the entire developmental spectrum. An honours graduate of UCD, from where she also obtained an MSc and PhD, she is a chartered psychologist, registered family therapist and supervisor, a member of both the Irish Council for Psychotherapy and the European Association for Psychotherapy, as well as the APA American Psychological Association and a former member of the Heads of Psychology Services in Ireland. Key clinical posts have included being Director of Psychology in St Vincent's Psychiatric Hospital Dublin and Director of Student Counselling Services in UCD. Marie served on the Medical Council of Ireland (2008–13) and on the Council of the Psychological Society of Ireland (2014–17). She has presented internationally, from the Tavistock and Portman NHS Trust in London to Peking University, Beijing. She was an *Irish Times* columnist for eight years and has been author, co-author, contributor and editor to a number of bestselling books, many with accompanying RTÉ radio programmes. Her appointment as Series Editor to the Cork University Press *MindYourSelf* series gathers a lifetime of professional experience to bring safe clinical information to general and professional readers.

CONTENTS

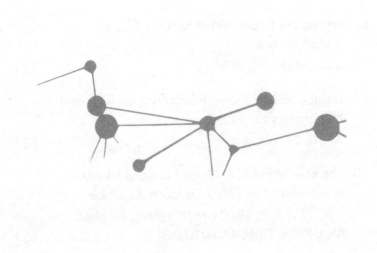

DISCLAIMER

This book has been written for general readers to introduce the topic or to increase their knowledge and understanding of it. It is not intended, or implied, to be a substitute for professional consultation or advice in this, or allied, areas. Any content, text, graphics, images or other information provided in any of the *MindYourSelf* books is for general purposes only.

On topics that have medical, psychological, psychiatric, psychotherapy, nursing, physiotherapy, occupational therapy, educational, vocational, organisational, sociological, legal or any mental health- or physical health-related or other content, *MindYourSelf* books do not replace diagnosis, treatment, or any other appropriate professional consultations and interventions. This also applies to any information or website links contained in the book.

While every effort has been made to ensure the accuracy of the information in the book, it is possible that errors or omissions may occur. Research also leads to new multidisciplinary perspectives in all professional areas, so that, despite all the publishers' caution and care, new thinking on certain topics may alter the accuracy of the content. The authors, editors and publishers can, therefore, assume no responsibility, nor provide any guarantees or warranties, concerning the up-to-date nature of the information provided.

MindYourSelf

Few expressions convey as much care as that lovely phrase 'mind yourself'. Quintessentially Irish, it is a blessing, an injunction, an endearment and a solicitous farewell. Like many simple phrases, 'mind yourself' has layers of psychological meaning, so that, while it trips lightly off the tongue at the end of conversations, there are depths of kindness that accompany it.

Being told to 'mind yourself' touches the heart. It resonates with the longing in each of us to have somebody in our world who cares about us. Saying 'mind yourself' means 'you matter to me', that what happens to you is important, and may nothing bad befall you. It is a cautionary phrase, with a gentle acknowledgement of your personal responsibility in self-care. Although it has become so ingrained in our leave-taking that we may not consciously note it, unconsciously, being minded is an atavistic need in all of us. 'Mind yourself' is what parents say to children, to adolescents, what people say to each other, to family and friends. We also say it to reassure ourselves that we have reminded those we love to keep themselves safe.

It is in this spirit of recognising the importance of self-care that the *MindYourSelf* book series has been designed; to bring safe, researched, peer-reviewed information from front-line professionals to help people to mind themselves. While, at one level, information – about everything – is now on multiple platforms at the touch of a screen, relying on internet sites is a problem. What is true? Who can you trust? How do you sift through the data to find what you need to know? Because it is not lack of access to facts, but fact overload, that makes people increasingly conscious of the dangers of misinformation, contradictory perspectives, internet prognoses, and the risk of unreliable or exploitative sources. What people want is simply the information that is relevant to them, delivered by professionals who care about their specialities and who are keen to help readers understand the topic. May this Cork University Press *MindYourSelf* series find its way to all who need it, and give readers the tools and resources to really mind themselves.

Dr Marie Murray, Series Editor, *MindYourSelf*

NOTES ON CONTRIBUTORS

Professor Peter Bede is the medical patron of the IMNDA; he is a consultant neurologist and professor in Trinity College Dublin. He leads a research group focusing on the pathological and imaging features of motor neurone disease and fronto-temporal dementia. With his team, he collaborates closely with international partners in France, the UK and Canada to develop accurate diagnostic, prognostic and monitoring protocols for clinical trials in MND. Peter holds a number of prestigious research grants from national and international funding agencies. His vision is to translate emerging academic insights to viable therapeutic strategies.

Dr Síle Carney is a psychologist who recently completed her research doctorate under the co-supervision of Professor Orla Hardiman and Dr Niall Pender. During her research she looked at the needs of caregivers supporting people with MND and sat at kitchen tables across Ireland listening to and recording caregivers' stories. Síle is committed to caregivers' voices getting heard and enabling them to access the support they need. She is currently training at the University of Limerick to become a clinical psychologist. Síle's interests centre on the use of research to help inform the development and provision of relevant supports for family caregivers.

Bernie Corr is the Beaumont hospital motor neurone disease clinical nurse specialist. She joined Professor Orla Hardiman's team in 1996. She was chairperson of the IMNDA and provided a nursing consultancy service. She won the HRB Junior Clinician Scientist Award, which facilitated a master's in science. As a member of the MND multidisciplinary team she provides an outreach service that is accessible and responsive to patients with MND, their families, the nurses in the IMNDA and members of the MDTs in hospices, hospitals and primary care facilities. She has a particular interest in respiratory and end-of-life management in MND.

Anne Corrigan is a barrister who leads the private client service in Arthur Cox. She is one of Ireland's leading authorities on trust law and charity law. Anne was lecturer in revenue law in the School of Law, UCD, from 1989 to 2000. She is a member of the Society of Trust and Estate Practitioners and co-author of *Trust and Succession Law* published by the Irish Taxation Institute. Anne has presented papers at numerous conferences on trust and taxation issues.

Róisín Duffy is the former chief executive of the Irish Motor Neurone Disease Association (IMNDA), the primary support organisation for people affected by MND. She has more than fifteen years' leadership experience in the not-for-profit sector and was responsible for the day-to-day financial management of the IMNDA and for developing and delivering on the association's long-term strategic goals. Throughout her time as CEO Róisín was committed to advocating on behalf of people affected by MND and she worked closely with other disability organisations and medical professionals around the country to ensure continuity of care.

Professor Orla Hardiman is professor of neurology at Trinity College Dublin and consultant neurologist at Beaumont hospital, where she is director of the national MND service.

She is chair of the Trinity College Academic Unit of Neurology and was appointed as the first full professor of neurology in 2014. She is the HSE national clinical lead in neurology, a founder of the European Treatment Initiative to Cure ALS (www.tricals.org), co-chair of the European Network for the Cure of ALS (ENCALS) and editor-in-chief of the journal *Amyotrophic Lateral Sclerosis and Frontotemporal Degeneration*.

Tracy Hutchin has played a pivotal role within the IMNDA since 2007 and in 2014 she was appointed as services manager. During her time with the association, Tracy has been a member of a number of working groups and steering committees working closely with organisations such as the Irish Hospice Foundation, the Neurological Alliance of Ireland (NAI), the Disability Federation of Ireland (DFI), Enable Ireland and the National Rehabilitation Hospital. Tracy coordinates and oversees the IMNDA services team and department, ensuring that we are always providing the highest-quality equipment and supports to our MND community.

Maeve Leahy is the public relations and communications executive of the IMNDA, to which position she was appointed in 2014. For a number of years prior to that she played an essential role within the organisation and has always been forthright and passionate about putting the voice of the MND client at the forefront of the association. Maeve works tirelessly to raise awareness of motor neurone disease and believes that the MND community deserves to be provided with the most accurate and up-to-date information.

Dr Stacey Li Hi Shing is a member of the Beaumont multidisciplinary ALS team and the Computational Neuroimaging Group in Trinity College Dublin. She is a medical graduate of Trinity College Dublin and she is currently pursuing a PhD on low-incidence motor neurone disease phenotypes. Her main research interest is the development of advanced imaging protocols to compare the radiological profile of motor neurone disease subgroups. She has published extensively on imaging signatures of ALS, PLS and poliomyelitis survivors. Her research contributed to the characterisation of compensatory brain changes, which is a new frontier of MND research.

Dr Jasmin Lope is a senior research fellow of the Computational Neuroimaging Group in Trinity College Dublin. She is a consultant child and adolescent psychiatrist, with a strong research interest in the neuroanatomical underpinnings of clinical disability. She is a medical graduate of Trinity College Dublin and a member of the UK Royal College of Psychiatrists. Her current research centres on complex computational radiological analyses to decipher the imaging correlates of common clinical manifestations. She has considerable clinical experience in the management of complex cases and a passion for service development.

Johanna McGrath is the information and support officer at the IMNDA. Her role revolves around providing information, advice and advocacy services to people with motor neurone disease, their families and caregivers. She liaises closely with the MND nurses and acts in an advisory capacity to the multidisciplinary team involved with the MND community.

Andy Minogue from Nenagh, County Tipperary, joined the civil service shortly after completing secondary school. He rose to senior management in Revenue. Unfortunately, he had to leave there in 2016 having been diagnosed with MND in 2015. He lived in Ardnacrusha, County Clare, with his wife Clare and their two teenage sons, Eoin and James. Andy sadly passed away in July 2021 having lived nobly and courageously with motor neurone disease.

Dr Ailín O'Dea is a senior clinical psychologist based in Beaumont hospital who has worked with people with physical illness for many years. She is currently engaged in research with Professor Orla Hardiman and Dr Niall Pender on support groups for caregivers of people with MND. Ailín has a particular interest in what helps people live as well as possible with life-limiting conditions. She is curious about mindfulness, spirituality and the role of the arts in coping with physical illness. She believes in collaborative research with patients and families. Ailín has personal experience of caring for loved ones with neurological conditions.

Dr Niall Pender is head of the Department of Psychology and principal clinical neuropsychologist at Beaumont hospital, Dublin, since 2003. He is associate professor in neuropsychology at Trinity College Dublin and honorary clinical associate professor at the Royal College of Surgeons in Ireland. Prior to this he was consultant neuropsychologist and clinical lead of the neuro-behavioural rehabilitation unit at the Royal Hospital for Neuro-disability, London. Niall is chair of the board of Headway and is a member of the boards of the

Motor Neurone Disease Research Foundation, and the Neurological Alliance of Ireland.

Dr Marta Pinto-Grau holds a PhD in neuropsychology and is currently completing her clinical psychology training at University College Dublin and the Health Service Executive. Marta completed an honours bachelor's degree in psychology at the University of Barcelona, and afterwards she completed a three-year master's degree in clinical neuropsychology at the Autonomous University of Barcelona. Marta then worked on the MND research team in Trinity College Dublin for seven years, where she completed her PhD. Her thesis examined neuropsychological phenotypes in people suffering from ALS and her work also explored how neuropsychological changes in ALS contribute to caregiver burden.

Dr Mary Rabbitte is the research programme manager at the All Ireland Institute of Hospice and Palliative Care. She previously worked as an accredited clinical psychotherapist with people with MND and their families within hospice and private practice and lectured on psychological rehabilitation in UCD. She has published research on psychotherapeutic approaches for people with MND and developed a national programme to improve psychosocial care with the IMNDA, Beaumont hospital and Our Lady's Hospice and Care Services funded by the Irish Hospice Foundation. Mary holds an MSc in counselling and psychotherapy from DCU and a PhD in chemistry from NUIG and has worked within the multinational sector with Ericsson.

Fidelma Rutledge has been an MND nurse with the IMNDA since 2007. She qualified as a general nurse in 1995 from the Whittington hospital in conjunction with the University of North London. She worked for two years in the National Hospital for Neurology and Neurosurgery, Queen Square, London, before returning to Ireland in 1997 and working in neurology at Beaumont hospital for nine years and completing a specialist practice course in neuroscience nursing.

Margaret Winters is a palliative care nurse with over twenty-five years' experience working in this speciality. She qualified in general nursing in Drogheda in 1989. Her interest in palliative care began when she worked in the Channel Islands. Further specialised training followed in the Northern Ireland Hospice in Belfast and the Royal Marsden hospital in London. Margaret has worked in a hospice inpatient unit, as part of a community palliative care team, and in hospice day services. She currently works as a clinical nurse manager in St Francis Hospice, Dublin, where her role includes working with patients and families coping with a life-limiting illness.

FOREWORD

Every two days someone on the island of Ireland is diagnosed with motor neurone disease (MND), which is a neurodegenerative condition in which the nerves that control voluntary muscles stop working. This means that messages gradually stop reaching the muscles, which leads to weakness and wasting that affects all the ordinary everyday activities that we take for granted, influencing how we walk, talk, eat, drink and breathe. *Living with Motor Neurone Disease: A complete guide* is designed to help anyone diagnosed with the disease, their family and friends to navigate their way through the progressive complexities that living with MND poses for everyone.

While MND is a rare disease, it is a devastating diagnosis. Life is altered unutterably and forever. MND when it strikes is ruthless, relentless and irreversible as it gradually and inexorably erodes capacities. It is a life-limiting condition that has no cure, with a trajectory that strikes initial terror into the hearts of those who are diagnosed with it, as many people so poignantly describe using terms such as 'an assassin', 'a thief', 'being in a nightmare', 'nothing but numbness', and 'facing the grim reaper'. Yet paradoxically, *Living with Motor Neurone Disease: A complete guide* is a book about hope rather than despair. It is positive, optimistic, practical and reassuring. It highlights ongoing research, for example 'the longest-running register of MND in the world is the Irish one, which is recognised internationally as one of the best of its kind'. It shows the exceptional strides being made to understand the subtypes of the disease; to track MND in origin and variability, in genetic and environmental interplay, in its commonalities and its exceptions and to decode and defeat it. As the fundraising

1

movement to support research into MND called 'Watch Your Back MND' (http://watchyourbackmnd.com) so powerfully proclaims, the fight against MND is on!

Living with Motor Neurone Disease: A complete guide is proud to be a part of that 'fight'. Written in collaboration with the Irish Motor Neurone Disease Association (IMNDA) by many of the most distinguished Irish experts on the condition, it is a book that shows the extraordinary power of multidisciplinary professionals working together in shared endeavour to support people diagnosed with MND and their carers. It is a guide on how to live *with* MND with the highest quality of life that is possible for as long as possible. Given the variability of the disease, that may be for a short time or for a long time, the classic example being Stephen Hawking, theoretical physicist, cosmologist and author, who lived for over half a century after his diagnosis with MND.

Research shows how having accurate information and timely access to services including doctors, neurologists, neuropsychologists, occupational therapists, speech therapists, physiotherapists, dieticians, respiratory physicians and local community healthcare professionals makes all the difference when it comes to a person's sense of control when living with MND. For this reason *Living with Motor Neurone Disease: A complete guide* is designed to be a step-by-step guide for *everyone*. It explains what MND is; how it is diagnosed and managed; how it affects the individual and the family; the psychological dimensions of the condition; the caregiver experience; living *with* the condition and facing the future too. It shows how to talk to children and adolescents, how to tell family and friends, how to adapt working conditions and home life. It describes all the supports available – medical, psychological, mechanical, technological and practical – to help cope with the daily impact of living with MND, particularly the essential supports provided and coordinated by the IMNDA.

When you open this book you tap into the combined expertise of clinicians across all aspects of MND, with each chapter addressing a different dimension. The 'Introduction' by the former CEO of the IMNDA Róisín Duffy sets the context by describing the ethos and activities of the association, which has been supporting people diagnosed with motor neurone disease and their families since 1985. Having collaborated with the IMNDA for the past two years on this book and learnt about their work, there are insufficient superlatives to describe what the IMNDA provides in kind and practical care – all based on its maxim 'until there is a cure, there is care'.

One of the most eminent internationally recognised authorities on MND, Professor Orla Hardiman, in her chapter 'What Is Motor Neurone Disease?' describes types of MND; causes and frequency within populations; and classification and prognosis based on when, where and how the first symptoms occur. She outlines potential personality changes and genetic and environmental factors that increase or decrease risk for any group of individuals. This is the ideal opening chapter because it details the complexity of MND but with reassurance from Professor Hardiman that, despite MND's 'very bad reputation', there are already positive indications (http://www.rmn.ie) about personalised medicine-based clinical trials to ensure 'the right patient will get the right drug, at the right time, in the right dose'.

Amongst those clinical scientists and researchers is the medical patron of the IMNDA Professor Peter Bede, who with Dr Stacey Li Hi Shing and Dr Jasmin Lope describes how early

3

symptoms of MND are often very subtle, occasional and non-specific and may therefore be mistaken for other conditions. 'Intermittent falls, clumsy hands, slurred speech after a long day, muscle twitching and coughing fits are not uncommon many months before the possibility of the diagnosis is even raised', so that the protracted diagnostic journey is not a reflection on any person or system but 'the inherent nature of any slowly progressive neurodegenerative condition'. This chapter is essential reading for anyone who wishes to understand the diagnostic and management process of MND or to learn more about the extensive research being conducted in the quest for further understanding of the condition.

In her chapter 'How Will Motor Neurone Disease Affect Me?' clinical nurse specialist Bernie Corr addresses the profound impact of a diagnosis of MND on a person and that person's family. Yet her chapter is one of reassurance about symptom relief, promotion of autonomy, crisis avoidance, maintaining independence as long as possible and enhancing quality of life. She affirms the importance of multidisciplinary care as she explains the symptoms that people may encounter but more importantly the interventions to help them when they do.

Information on the extent to which changes in thinking and behaviour may occur is addressed in Chapter 4 by neuropsychologists Dr Niall Pender and Dr Marta Pinto-Grau. Emphasising that while cognitive and behavioural changes are not inevitable, in extreme instances changes may include disinhibition, impulsivity, anger, irritability, physical or verbally aggressive behaviour and lack of empathy. There may be uncontainable involuntary laughing or crying which is distressing for the person with MND and those around them. Strategies for managing behavioural difficulties and ways of understanding how 'these difficulties reflect the effects of changes in the sufferer's brain and are not intentional or deliberate' are offered with compassionate clinical expertise to support the person, family members and especially carers so that caretaker burden is alleviated and appropriate help can be given to everyone.

In their chapter 'How Will Motor Neurone Disease Affect My Family?' psychotherapist Dr Mary Rabbitte and psychologist Dr Síle Carney address the big questions that arise at the moment of diagnosis: 'Is this really so?' 'Could there be a mistake?' 'How will I tell the people I love?' Then there are the questions children ask: 'Can I catch it too?' 'What will happen to you?' 'Will you die?' With recognition of the impact on different family members depending on their age and their development stage at the time a parent is diagnosed, the chapter is rich with tips on how to talk about MND, and how to cope with role reversals, altered family dynamics, increased caretaking, and family life.

Life is exceptionally challenging for those who find themselves in the caretaker role, as Chapter 6 on 'The Caregiver Experience' by psychologists Dr Ailín O'Dea and Dr Síle Carney explains. Opening their chapter with the caregiver quote *My father didn't get a diagnosis of MND, our whole family did*, they emphasise the importance of 'carers' caring for themselves so they do not become distressed, depleted or burnt out.

Perhaps the most poignant chapter in this book is that of Andy Minogue, who was diagnosed with motor neurone disease in 2015. In Chapter 7 he generously shared his personal experience of living with MND in accordance with the BATTLE HARD approach he devised. Sadly Andy died in July 2021 before the publication of this book but his words will live on forever.

One of the misconceptions of palliative care is that it is not introduced until the final stages of a person's life, but, as Margaret Winters in her sensitive chapter 'Facing the Future: What to expect from palliative care' points out, palliative care is concerned with quality of life from the moment of diagnosis, with psychosocial support for everyone 'every step of the way'. Supportive too is the wealth of information provided in Chapter 9 by barrister Anne Corrigan on 'Legal Considerations: Information on wills and managing your assets'. This also addresses issues such as general and enduring power of attorney, trusts and taxes and the importance of timely consultation with one's solicitor for future planning. Finally, Chapter 10 on 'The Role of the Irish Motor Neurone Disease Association and Other Supports Available' is a must-read as it provides an exceptionally comprehensive account of services and supports provided through the IMNDA.

Anyone who has been a carer for someone they love knows how fulfilling and rewarding, demanding and exhausting, emotionally torturous, achingly lonely and socially isolating it can be. They know how it can arouse ambivalent feelings of empathy and anger, guilt and grief, pity and indifference, tenderness and the terror of being unable to continue with fear of burnout and compassion fatigue. They know that sometimes caring is the most precious and profound life experience, while at other times it can annihilate with the sadness and sorrow of witnessing the incremental losses suffered by someone you love and the anticipatory grief at their dwindling capabilities and increased dependency, which evokes the inevitable unanswerable question, 'Why?'

My experience of editing *Living with Motor Neurone Disease: A complete guide* is: what a privilege it has been to do so. It has been profoundly moving, hugely instructive and extraordinarily edifying as I have learnt about the world of MND and the resilience of those who have received a diagnosis, the professionals who support them, the families who care for them, the researchers who seek a solution (www.rmn.ie) and the exceptional way in which people live their lives with MND (https://www.youtube.com/watch?v=P9tSlqQSCXE) and fight to fundraise and help others who will come after them (www. wwyc.ie).

May this book now find its way to all who need it and may the sales be many, so that the royalties, all of which are dedicated to the IMNDA, will help towards funding services and research for MND.

Dr Marie Murray, Editor, and Series Editor *MindYourSelf*

ACKNOWLEDGEMENTS

We are very grateful for the support of many individuals during the preparation of this volume. In particular, we want to thank Dr Marie Murray, Editor of this book and *MindYourSelf* Series Editor, for her outstanding support and belief in this project. This volume would never have seen the light of day if it wasn't for Marie's expertise, drive, determination and enthusiasm.

We would also like to thank all at Cork University Press, especially Mike Collins, Publications Director; Maria O'Donovan, Editor; Aonghus Meaney and Alison Burns.

The IMNDA also wishes to acknowledge the wonderful support of our former Chief Executive Officer Róisín Duffy, without whose leadership and direction we would have been lost during this and many other projects. She has been our committed captain who has steadied the boat through many a storm. We will miss her greatly as she takes on other projects but we will always be grateful to her.

The IMNDA must also acknowledge the immediate response to this publishing venture and the incredible input of Maeve Leahy and all the team, particularly Johanna McGrath, Fidelma Rutledge and Tracy Hutchin, who immersed themselves in this project to bring information on motor neurone disease to further public and professional attention.

There are so many people who played a part in the development of this work. We are deeply indebted to the generosity of all the experts who work at the coalface of MND research and clinical management who gave up their valuable time and committed to this guide. Their contributions provide vital information that will benefit not only people living with motor neurone disease and their families and friends but also health-care professionals.

Perhaps the most significant contribution in this book is that of Andy Minogue, who was diagnosed with motor neurone disease in 2015 and who has not lived to see his words in print. Andy you imprinted yourself in our minds and hearts and we are most grateful to you for all you did to create awareness of MND.

We must pay particular tribute to the late Fr Tony Coote, who was the inspiration for this book. Thank you, Tony, your memory continues to motivate us, implores us to strive for better, and encourages us to do what we can while we can.

Finally, our sincerest thanks must go to all our MND community – to all those living with the disease and their families – this book is for you.

INTRODUCTION

Irish Motor Neurone Disease Association

Róisín Duffy

Navigating your way through a complex condition such as motor neurone disease (MND) can be stressful at the best of times and debilitating at the worst. Throw a complex, under-pressure and bureaucratic healthcare system into the mix and it becomes a minefield.

It is my hope that this book will offer not only comfort and reassurance to everyone affected by MND, but that it will also be an invaluable resource that will inform, educate, prepare and signpost people to a range of both practical everyday supports and clinical expertise.

The Irish Motor Neurone Disease Association (IMNDA) has cared for and supported people living with motor neurone disease and their families since 1985. Over the years, we have grown, adapted and changed course many times but one thing has remained steadfast, and that is our commitment to person-centred care. We are privileged to work closely with our medical colleagues in both hospital and community settings around the country to deliver this joined-up care.

There is no 'one size fits all' when it comes to motor neurone disease. No two journeys are the same, and it is with this in mind that the association tailors its core supports. We have seen first-hand how an MND diagnosis can send a family into a tailspin. For many, it could be the first time they have heard the words 'motor neurone disease' and the fear of the unknown can be extremely stressful. I have heard the expression 'we all got the diagnosis' on more than one occasion and I think this sums up the emotional rollercoaster accurately. It is very definitely a family affair when it comes to dealing with the diagnosis and the disease and that is why it is so important that a holistic approach is applied, taking everyone's needs into consideration.

Having information and access to the best available services including doctors, neurologists, MND outreach nurses and local community healthcare professionals makes all the difference when it comes to a person's journey with MND. As does being registered with the Irish Motor Neurone Disease Association and having access to its everyday practical supports.

Dealing with the reality of MND is not only about knowing the answers, it is about knowing the questions you need to ask and who you need to speak to in order to get the correct answers. That is why one of the most invaluable services offered by the IMNDA is our outreach MND nursing service. Upon registering, each family is appointed a designated nurse who will remain their main point of contact for the duration of the disease. This nurse will liaise with other medical professionals on your care team, including local healthcare professionals, to ensure an appropriate care pathway is put in place from the start. They will also keep you updated about the various services available to you through the IMNDA. We know how important it is for everyone to understand what options of care and support are available to them, especially when it comes to everyday living and future-proofing your life and your environment.

Ireland's population has grown hugely over the last number of years and so too has the number of people who are registered with IMNDA and under our care. According to the Central Statistics Office's *Population and Labour Force*

Projections 2017–2051, Ireland's population is expected to grow by approximately 60,000 people every year for the next ten years. If this transpires, in ten years' time it estimates there will be more people aged over sixty-five than under fourteen. The peak age of onset of MND in Ireland is around sixty-three.

More people means more demand, which is why it is so important that we as an organisation work closely with governing bodies in the years ahead to ensure that adequate healthcare initiatives are in place so that people living with MND can live as active, independent citizens in their own homes for as long as possible. This is one of the IMNDA's top priorities, which aligns with the Department of Health's long-term Sláintecare Action Plan – Right Care. Right Time. Right Place.

Having a proactive approach to care is paramount when it comes to MND. We in the Irish Motor Neurone Disease Association work hard to deliver the everyday support that's needed to keep people at home with their loved ones. As well as providing an outreach nursing team who travel the country visiting people, the IMNDA also supplies crucial mobility aids and equipment and life-changing communication aids on loan to every person who needs them. Having equipment such as specialised beds, powered wheelchairs, hoists and riser recliners as and when needed ensures people living with MND can remain independent in their own homes for as long as possible. The right equipment also helps to alleviate some of the burden of care often felt by families and primary caregivers.

In the last few years, we have seen an increase in the number of people availing of our counselling grant. Finding ways to cope following an MND diagnosis can be incredibly difficult for families and not everyone will process the diagnosis in the same way, or at the same time. The value of talking to a trained professional cannot be underestimated and can often be the difference between coping and not coping. So for those who want to talk, I would strongly encourage it, as many of our community have told us it was a great source of comfort to be able to articulate their worst fears and to have them allayed as far as possible in a safe and confidential environment.

Another vital service provided by the IMNDA is our home care grant. The association provides financial assistance towards extra home care hours when there is a shortfall in what is needed versus what the Health Service Executive (HSE) can provide. Funding cuts in certain pockets of the country has often resulted in lengthy time lags between application and receipt of home care hours, which is why the IMNDA's grant is so important. Once a carer is available through one of our partner home care providers, those hours can be actioned quickly. The power of a few extra hours can never be underestimated as it gives everyone in the family that extra care and support, whether it be respite for a family member or additional personal care for the person living with MND.

Recognising that today's research could be tomorrow's treatment and cures, we are proud to have strong links with Professor Orla Hardiman and her team of researchers in Trinity College Dublin. Providing funding for both national and international research projects into the causes of the disease, better treatments, and one day hopefully a cure is another one of our main priorities. With every new study or clinical trial there are learnings, developments and breakthroughs – and with this comes hope. We need to remain hopeful. We are also privileged to be able to fund a research fellow post in Trinity College. The ultimate aim of all services provided and all research projects funded through the IMNDA is to improve the lives of people living with MND and their families, and words cannot express our gratitude to those who give of themselves, their time, their talents or financial aid on behalf of those who are living with motor neurone disease.

At this time of transition from being CEO of the Irish Motor Neurone Disease Association to being former CEO, among the many projects that I have been privileged to support is this significant book, *Living with Motor Neurone Disease: A complete guide*, which I believe will give readers greater insight into MND. While the complexity of the disease means that not all the answers we would wish to give can be given, and while no cure is yet available, with this book we hope to convey the deep commitment of the IMNDA to the lives of all who receive a diagnosis of motor neurone disease. Perhaps this will also open up important conversations about MND.

Until there is a cure, there is care. The Irish Motor Neurone Disease Association will always be here to offer care and support to every person who needs it.

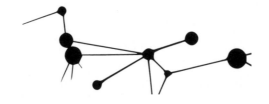

CHAPTER 1

What Is Motor Neurone Disease?

PROFESSOR ORLA HARDIMAN

INTRODUCTION

Motor neurone disease (MND), also known as Lou Gehrig disease and Amyotrophic lateral sclerosis (ALS), is a progressive neurological condition in which the nerves that control voluntary muscles stop working.

Motor neurones are nerve cells that control voluntary movement. The nervous system is very complex, and the intricate circuitry of movement is not fully understood. But we know that nerves that control movement can be roughly divided into two categories – those that originate in the brain and send projections (axons) through the white matter down to the spinal cord; and those that sit in the spinal cord and send out projections or messages to muscles.

The upper motor neurones are located mainly in the grey matter on the outer surface of the brain. These neurones are sometimes called Betz cells, or pyramidal cells. Messages from these neurones make their way down to the spinal cord. They pass electrical signals through various 'relay stations' that help to make voluntary movements smooth and accurate. These axons then connect through chemical signalling to the nerves in the spinal cord.

The lower motor neurones reside in the spinal cord (in the front middle part of the spinal cord, to be exact, in a location called the 'anterior horn') and project to the muscle. These motor neurones are sometimes called anterior horn cells because of their location. For this reason, MND is sometimes called 'anterior horn cell disease' by neurologists. Anterior horn neurones send electrical signals through their projections to all muscles that are under voluntary control, including those of the trunk, limbs, and the muscles controlling speech and swallowing, and those controlling breathing. 'Involuntary' muscles like those of the gut, heart, bladder and bowels have a different type of nerve supply.

For 'voluntary' muscles to work properly, they need an intact nerve supply. We know that when the nerve supply to the muscle is damaged, the muscle becomes irritable, and begins to lose its bulk. If the nerve supply is impaired but not completely disrupted, small parts of the muscle can become unstable and begin to twitch. Sometimes these twitches, which are called fasciculations, can be seen in muscles close to the skin. People with early motor neurone disease can also develop cramping for the same reason.

It is important to realise that cramping and fasciculations also occur in normal people. Fasciculations can be caused by stress, caffeine and some medications. Some people develop cramps and fasciculations for no apparent reason – a condition called benign fasciculation syndrome. This can be distressing but does not develop into MND.

When upper motor neurones stop working, the control of movement is interrupted. The effect is increased muscle stiffness (spasticity) and impaired fine movements (like fastening buttons, inserting a key into a lock, or managing zips). This is also what happens when a person has a stroke. When lower motor neurones stop working, the muscles lose their nerve supply and cannot contract properly. This leads to thinning of muscles (wasting) and marked weakness with prominent muscle fasciculations or twitches.

Because MND can lead to degeneration of *both* upper and lower motor neurones, the condition is associated with muscle wasting, fasciculations, weakness, and enhanced reflexes. There are very few other conditions that have this combination of upper *and* lower motor neurone degeneration. In MND the sensory system is usually not affected and people with MND don't describe loss of sensation or pins and needles (paraesthesia). Because MND is mainly a disorder of voluntary muscles, the muscles of the heart and the digestive system are not affected. The bladder is sometimes affected later in the illness, but bowel control is unaffected.

Types of MND: ALS, PLS and PMA

Most people with MND experience a combination of upper and lower motor neurone degeneration. In Ireland, this accounts for around 90 per cent of people we see with the condition, and is sometimes termed amyotrophic lateral sclerosis (ALS). However, there are a number of very rare forms of the condition in which there is exclusive involvement of upper motor neurones, or exclusive involvement of lower motor neurones.

When the upper motor neurones alone are involved, the condition is called primary lateral sclerosis (PLS). This condition is rare and is difficult to diagnose in the early stages. Most experts like to wait at least four years before they can be certain of the diagnosis. Similarly, those who have exclusive involvement of the lower motor neurones may have a condition called progressive muscular atrophy (PMA). This is also very rare, and it can be difficult to be certain about the diagnosis. Both PLS and PMA carry a better prognosis (or likely course or outcome) than typical MND (ALS).

Some people have exclusive involvement of their speech and swallowing muscles, a condition called progressive bulbar palsy. This is also very rare and occurs mostly in older women, for reasons that are not fully understood.

Spinal versus bulbar-onset MND

Motor neurone disease is sometimes classified based on where the first symptom occurs.

For example, if the nerves supplying muscles in the arms, legs or trunk are affected first, it is described as 'spinal onset'. Conversely, if the nerves supplying muscles of speech or swallow are affected first, it is described as 'bulbar onset'.

Spinal onset is more common in men, and bulbar onset is more common in older women. Some people with MND (around 5 per cent) begin with problems catching their breath, and with difficulty lying down flat. This usually points to involvement of the diaphragm, and is termed 'respiratory onset'.

Changes in thinking and behaviour

Although we originally thought that MND was a condition that only affected the motor system, we know now that up to 50 per cent of people will also experience some changes in thinking and behaviour. This is very severe in around 15 per cent of cases. In those affected, there is evidence of problems in multitasking, and in making decisions that require complex planning. A high proportion of these individuals also experience changes in their personality and behaviour. These symptoms can be very distressing for caregivers and family members.

How frequent is MND?

The frequency of MND is relatively consistent within populations of European extraction. Around one person in thirty thousand develops MND in each year. In Ireland, on average, this amounts to around 150 new diagnoses every year.

The prevalence of MND (the number of cases at any given time) is around one person in twelve thousand, amounting to about 350 cases at any one time in Ireland. There is no reason to believe that MND is becoming more common in Ireland, once we correct for the changes in structure and size in the Irish population. The overall rates (per 100,000) have remained the same over the past 25 years, although the total number of people in Ireland with MND has increased. This increase is related to the overall rise in the Irish population, and the larger numbers of older people in the population.

MND can strike at any age. However, the peak age of onset of MND in Ireland is around sixty-three. Men are slightly more likely to develop MND than women. The rates of MND in Ireland are similar to those in other European countries. But the rates of MND are not uniform across the world. We know that it is less common in some non-European populations, for example the rates are lower in Asia, and much lower in populations that are mixed, such as Latin America and the Caribbean. We don't know the reasons for this, but there is evidence that mixing genes from different ancestral groups may be protective.

What causes MND?

MND is definitely more than one condition, and probably has many different causes. We know that genetic susceptibility is important, and that this susceptibility probably combines with exposures within the environment to trigger the disease later in life. However, we don't know what these exposures are, nor do we know how they interact with the genetic risk factors.

In some people (in Ireland, approximately 15 per cent of those diagnosed with MND) another family member has also had motor neurone disease or an associated dementia (fronto-temporal dementia), suggesting a genetic cause for this type of MND. Over the past thirty years, at least thirty genes have been associated with an increased risk of developing MND. These genes vary in importance based on their frequency (or the rate at which they occur) within individual populations.

Only one of these known genes is important as a cause of MND in Ireland. This gene is called C9orf72, and it accounts for around 8–10 per cent of all cases of MND in Ireland. The motor neurone disease gene mutation in C9orf72 also causes dementia. Other disease-causing gene variants that are common in other countries (for example SOD1, which is frequent in the US) are not found in the Irish population.

We know that this gene called C9orf72 is also associated with other psychiatric conditions, and that other genetic factors that increase the risk for MND can also increase the risk for other neurological and psychiatric conditions within some families. For example, some families of people with MND who do not carry the abnormal C9orf72 gene variant also have higher than expected rates of psychosis and other psychological conditions. This overlap between MND and psychiatric conditions is also confirmed by detailed genetic studies. We have found a 14 per cent overlap in the risk for developing MND and schizophrenia. We do not yet know what these genes are or how they interact with other genes/environmental exposure to lead to one type of condition in one family member and another type in another family member.

Can we test for MND genes?

Genetic testing for some genes is possible in MND. In Ireland, this is really only relevant for the gene C9orf72. For people with MND who wish to be tested, we strongly recommend that they have a consultation with an expert in the genetics of MND, and that they receive counselling before and after the testing to make sure that they understand the implications of the results for themselves and their families. This is important because not everybody who carries a genetic risk will wish to know their genetic status, and people have an entitlement not to be tested if they do not wish to know whether they carry an abnormal gene. This should be made clear to the person with MND before testing takes place so that they have a choice.

It is also important to be aware that we do not know for definite whether the abnormal gene will always cause MND, and for this reason we do not recommend testing other family members who do not have symptoms, unless this takes place as part of a research programme. If participating in a research project, the family member should be provided with a detailed information leaflet about the research, and should sign a consent form showing that they understand the implications of their participation. However, it is also important to note that this approach might change in the future as new treatments become available.

Environmental causes of MND

There have been many studies on possible environmental exposures and MND, but none have been definitive. In Ireland detailed studies of MND over twenty-five years have not shown any real evidence of clustering in any part of the country. While there is some evolving evidence from other countries that exposure to some pollutants and pesticides might increase the risk of developing MND, this remains to be confirmed, and in any event, the risk is likely to be very small. In Ireland, when we correct for the number of people living in an area, there is no real difference in the frequency of MND in rural compared to urban areas, nor is there any real difference in disease frequency in industrialised compared to non-industrialised regions of the country.

There is some evidence that smoking might increase the risk of developing MND. Whether specific types of activities or occupations are associated with increased risk remains controversial. For example, we know that MND seems to be more common in some types of elite athletes, such as soccer and rugby players. But whether engaging in exercise of itself increases risk is not clear. Some studies show that gentle exercise might be beneficial, whereas others show that intense exercise increases risk. The likely explanation, although still unproven, is that the genetic factors that make a person both interested in exercise and also good at sports may also be the same genetic factors that increase the risk for developing MND. A very old study from the US also showed that those who developed MND later in life tended to be thinner and more likely to have engaged in sporting activities while in college. This also fits with some observations that people who are overweight and carry high risk for heart attacks and strokes may also be at lower risk for developing MND.

Part of the difficulty in establishing risk factors lies in the likelihood that MND is really a syndrome (a group of symptoms that occur together) rather than a single condition. For this reason, the relative importance of different exposures might also be determined by a person's genetic make-up. This is called a gene–environment interaction. We do not have enough information yet on the genetic factors that increase the risk of developing MND, nor do we know enough about likely environmental factors that truly increase the risk.

It is important to remember that motor neurone disease is a rare disease. The lifetime risk of developing MND in the Irish population is 1:300. This compares to the risk of developing a heart attack or a stroke, which is around 1:3. So finding risk factors that might interact with a person's genetic make-up will require very large studies of thousands of patients across many different countries. These studies are already under way within our European consortium, but it will take some time for us to develop a full understanding of the complexity of the disease and the different factors that increase or decrease risk for any group of individuals.

What happens to the motor neurones in MND?

We know that the motor neurones degenerate in MND, but exactly what is happening inside the cells is not well understood. There is evidence that the way the motor neurones manage certain proteins becomes impaired, and that some proteins form clumps (called misfolded protein) within the cells. Some scientists think that this type of protein misfolding can be damaging to cells, and that the damage spreads to the other neurones that connect with these damaged neurones, leading to the statement 'what wires together dies together'.

We also know that when neurones become damaged, the surrounding cells, some of which belong to the immune system, become activated and secrete chemicals that can lead to further damage to the neurones. This leads to a cascade of damage that then spreads to other parts of the motor system, leading to the symptoms of MND.

Much of the research that is under way in MND is focused on our understanding of what leads to the protein misfolding, how this spreads to other cells, and how the immune system becomes activated and contributes to the degeneration.

MND prognosis

MND has a very bad reputation. Receiving a diagnosis often feels like an immediate death sentence. While it is true that, for the vast majority of people, MND shortens life expectancy, there is huge variability and everybody's experience of the condition is different. Some people experience a very rapid progression, but a smaller percentage progress very slowly and can live for a very long time.

Ireland and some other countries in Europe including Holland, Italy, Scotland, England and Germany have maintained registers of MND. The longest-running register of MND in the world is the Irish one, which is recognised internationally as one of the best of its kind. Recently our research groups combined information from all of our European registers to try to predict prognosis. This is important when we are recruiting people to clinical trials, as we need to make sure that those receiving the test drug have the same prognosis as those receiving the dummy drug.

We have found that the factors that determine outcome (survival) include:

- age of onset (younger is better)
- site of onset (spinal is better)
- length of time from first symptom to diagnosis (longer is better)
- whether breathing is affected
- whether the person has lost a lot of weight
- whether thinking is affected
- whether the condition is associated with the C9orf72 gene variant (this carries a slightly worse prognosis).

However, it is important to remember that everybody is different, and while 70 per cent of people with MND tend to survive around three years from their first symptom, the remaining 30 per cent have a much longer life expectancy. Moreover, we should remember that interventions such as breathing support using non-invasive ventilation and attendance at a multidisciplinary clinic can enhance survival. Also new drugs aimed at slowing down disease progression are now being developed and tested in clinical trials.

Medications

There is no treatment that stops MND. However, most neurologists, MND clinics and healthcare professionals would prescribe riluzole, which has a modest effect in slowing down the disease. Other medications can be used to help with mood, muscle stiffness (spasticity), problems of uncontrollable laughter/crying (called pseudobulbar affect, which is a common feature of MND), increased amounts of saliva and drooling, and pain. Some people with MND and arm weakness also develop shoulder pain. This can be treated with shoulder injection and physiotherapy. In the later stages of the condition, the palliative care team often use opiate-based treatments, both for pain and to help with breathing-related symptoms.

Clinical trials and drug development

To date, the many advances in understanding the complexity of MND have not translated into effective therapies. However, this is changing. There are already clinical trials under way for some of the genetic forms of MND. In addition, as we increase our understanding of the subtypes of MND, there will be new personalised medicine-based clinical trials that will ensure that the right patient will get the right drug, at the right time, in the right dose.

Conclusions

The syndrome of MND is complex, and can no longer be viewed as a pure motor system degeneration. There are strong overlaps with other neurodegenerative conditions, notably frontotemporal dementia. Recent scientific advances have begun to uncover the complex processes involved in MND. And although effective treatments remain elusive, good clinical management can improve survival and quality of life.

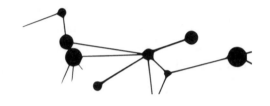

CHAPTER 2

The Diagnosis and Management of Motor Neurone Disease

DR STACEY LI HI SHING, DR JASMIN LOPE,
PROFESSOR PETER BEDE

Diagnostic considerations

The early diagnosis of motor neurone disease (MND) can be challenging and it often takes a number of visits to various specialists to establish the diagnosis. Early symptoms of MND are often very subtle, intermittent and non-specific and may therefore be attributed to fatigue or mistaken for other conditions. Intermittent falls, clumsy hands, slurred speech after a long day, muscle twitching and coughing fits are not uncommon many months before the possibility of the diagnosis is even raised.

The first point of contact is often the GP, who typically performs a thorough physical examination. Sometimes, no objective clinical findings can be identified early in the course of the disease. The average interval between the first symptoms and the definite diagnosis is around twelve months. The protracted diagnostic journey in MND is not a reflection on a specific healthcare system, geographical region, GP or neurologist, but rather the inherent nature of any slowly progressive neurodegenerative condition.

Compared to other neurological conditions, MND exhibits considerable variability in initial symptoms, disease progression rates and age of onset. It is not uncommon for MND-associated symptoms to be initially attributed to other conditions, such as carpal tunnel syndrome, slipped discs, and peripheral nerve problems, or it may even be mistaken for psychological issues at first. It is easy to criticise misdiagnoses in retrospect when the manifestations of MND are obvious, but as it is a rare disease, the initial consideration of more common conditions may be reasonable.

What happens after referral?

Once a referral is made to a neurologist, a systematic and structured approach is needed to confirm a suspected diagnosis as follows:

- a detailed clinical history

- family history

- medication history

- occupational history

- exposure to environmental factors

- physical and neurological examination.

These are all indispensable. Electrical, laboratory and radiological tests are not necessarily required to confirm the diagnosis of MND, but these are often undertaken to rule out alternative neurological diagnoses which may mimic MND. The specific tests recommended by the neurologist depend on the findings on examination and the constellation of initial symptoms.

Ruling out alternative diagnoses

Brain and spinal cord scans (MRI) are often helpful to rule out alternative structural or inflammatory processes, but they are not absolutely necessary.

- Patients with bulbar-onset disease are particularly likely to benefit from brain imaging.

- Spinal MRI is useful to rule out cord compression, tumours, vascular malformations, inflammatory changes, or the compression of spinal nerve roots. As many people suffer from some degree of back pain and protruding discs, clinical and radiological findings need to be carefully integrated. Depending on the initial symptoms, additional tests, such as blood tests and cerebrospinal fluid analyses from a spinal tap, may also be performed. The main role of these tests in suspected motor neurone disease is to rule out alternative diagnoses.

- Blood tests are useful to assess for systematic infections, autoimmune conditions, endocrine abnormalities, vitamin deficiencies, and malignancies.

- Spinal fluid analyses can also be helpful to reassuringly rule out central nervous system infections, malignancy or autoimmune conditions. Spinal taps are typically performed as an outpatient or day hospital procedure, sometimes under radiological (X-ray) guidance.

- Genetic testing is not required to establish the diagnosis of MND but can be helpful to confirm specific MND types such as Kennedy's disease (SBMA).

Confirming the diagnosis

'Electrical' tests (formally called 'neurophysiology' or 'electro-physiology' studies) are particularly helpful to evaluate affected muscles and nerves. These tests look at spontaneous electrical activity in the muscles suggestive of motor nerve degeneration.

Voluntary muscle activity is controlled by a two-tier command structure. The upper motor neurones (UMN) are located in the area of the brain called the 'motor cortex'. These neurones have very long tails (axons) that descend through a convoluted path into the brainstem and spinal cord. They interface with the lower motor neurones (LMN) that leave the spinal cord and make their way to specific muscles.

The assessment of the *upper motor neurone system* requires a very careful physical examination, focusing on muscle tone and various reflexes. Upper motor neurone signs include brisk reflexes, cramping, and muscle stiffness. The clinical manifestations of *lower motor neurone degeneration* include muscle wasting, twitching, and weakness. To establish the diagnosis of amyotrophic lateral sclerosis (ALS), one has to demonstrate that both the upper and lower motor neurone systems are affected. Neurologists typically distinguish between limb onset ('spinal-onset') and voice or swallowing onset ('bulbar-onset') forms of ALS.

While MND can be diagnosed by any neurologist, it is often helpful to see a neurologist with a special interest in neuromuscular disorders or someone who cares for many patients with MND. A second opinion is often sought, and there are cases when the diagnosis is suspected for a long time but formal electrophysiological or clinical criteria are not met.

Manifestations of the Disease

Bulbar manifestations of MND include slurred speech, coughing fits when eating or drinking, difficulty with crumbly foods, and tongue wasting. An unusual manifestation of the disease is what is called 'pseudobulbar affect' (PBA) or 'pathological crying and laughing' (PCL). This refers to uncontrollable crying or laughing, which is a distressing symptom. Patients with PBA may start tearing up watching an emotive TV commercial or start laughing excessively in situations which they don't find particularly amusing. These symptoms may cause embarrassment and may limit a person's social activities and lead to avoidance of public places. The recognition and discussion of PBA is very important as there are a number of medications which can bring these symptoms under control.

It cannot be emphasised enough that muscle twitching, slurred speech, muscle wasting and muscle stiffness can be caused by *many other medical and neurological conditions*, so the constellation of these symptoms does not necessarily suggest MND.

It is also noteworthy that the term 'MND' encompasses a multitude of syndromes which include:

- amyotrophic lateral sclerosis (ALS)

- Kennedy's disease (spinal and bulbar muscular atrophy: SBMA)

- primary lateral sclerosis (PLS)

- progressive muscular atrophy (PMA)

- spinal muscular atrophy (SMA)

- rare conditions such as Mills' syndrome

Primary lateral sclerosis (PLS) is associated with selective *upper motor neurone* (UMN) dysfunction, and people with PLS typically experience falls, lower limb stiffness and cramping. It carries a relatively good prognosis. It is however a particularly challenging diagnosis to establish because ALS can also present with predominant upper motor neurone signs initially.

Kennedy's disease is a genetic disorder involving the *lower motor neurone* system. It affects male patients and has a number of non-neurological manifestations in addition to weakness, muscle twitching and wasting.

It is important to carefully distinguish all these syndromes from ALS, because they are associated with different clinical outcomes and care needs. The medical terminology may be somewhat confusing, but the main message is that there are many types of motor neurone disease, each associated with a distinct set of symptoms, medical outcomes and specific management needs. Motor neurone disease is merely an umbrella term and patients with MND can have markedly different symptoms and care needs.

The multidisciplinary team

Once the diagnosis of MND is established, a thorough multidisciplinary assessment is required. Multidisciplinary MND clinics have been carefully set up to pre-empt, monitor and manage MND-associated symptoms. In MND care, a multidisciplinary team (MDT) typically consists of the following:

- an experienced MND specialist nurse

- a social worker

- a dietician

- a speech and language therapist

- an occupational therapist

- a physiotherapist

- a neuropsychologist

- a neurologist

- a neurophysiologist/electrophysiologist

- a respiratory physician

- an interventional radiologist for feeding tube insertions.

There is ample evidence that specialist MDT clinics provide effective, individualised management for a variety of presentations and disease variants. Given the relative rarity of MND compared to other neurological conditions, the contribution of experienced healthcare professionals to MND clinics is invaluable. The role of the multidisciplinary team is twofold: (1) screening for symptoms which may be associated with the disease and (2) the dynamic management of emerging symptoms.

Initial assessment

The initial MDT assessment would typically include a comprehensive evaluation for nutritional status, swallowing, speech, mobility, dexterity, muscle stiffness, respiratory function (breathing), cognition, and social support.

- Breathing can be assessed by pulmonary function tests (PFTs) or portable devices such as sniff nasal inspiratory pressure (SNIP) testing.

- Overnight oxygen levels can be monitored by a finger-clipped device called a pulse oximeter, which helps to identify dips in oxygen levels non-invasively.

- Nutritional status, diet and weight loss are carefully monitored and patients with swallowing difficulties may need feeding tube placement to maintain their weight. The optimal timing of feeding tube insertion requires experience and careful coordination between multidisciplinary team members.

Supportive interventions for independence

The governing concept behind any supportive intervention in MND is to maintain independence and adapt to existing lifestyles, while maintaining dignity and autonomy. Dietetic, respiratory and mobility interventions are tailored to individual care needs, so they can be implemented in the patient's community, home environment, during travel or at work.

Maintaining mobility and reducing fall risk is an important aspect of preserving independence. While some patients suffer from weak ankles ('foot drop'), wrists ('wrist drop') or neck ('head drop'), others suffer from considerable stiffness in their limbs and joints. Depending on individual symptom profiles, personalised assistive devices such as walking aids, ankle-foot orthoses (AFOs), wrist splints, wheelchairs, chin lifts, or stair lifts help to assure safety at home and prevent falls.

Monitoring respiration

Another key aspect of MND care revolves around the careful monitoring for respiratory insufficiency. Breathing problems may present as:

- early-morning headaches

- exercise intolerance

- unexplained fatigue

- recurrent chest infections

- difficulty clearing secretions.

Respiratory management typically centres on the introduction of non-invasive ventilation (NIV) which can be used overnight, or during the day as needed. These machines provide a pre-set pressure via a facial mask to help breathing and synchronise with the patient's natural respiratory cycles. It often takes some time to get used to these machines, but most patients tolerate them well and report significantly improved energy levels. These machines are relatively light and portable.

Managing fatigue

Fatigue is a common symptom of MND, which is likely to stem from a combination of factors, owing to respiratory compromise, medications, nutritional deficits, poor sleep, discomfort, low mood and possibly disease-specific metabolic changes. It is important to carefully review these factors and adjust medications if necessary to reduce fatigue. Sleep is often fragmented in ALS, something that also needs to be discussed with the MND multidisciplinary team. Discomfort from muscle aches, pain in pressure areas, difficulty synchronising with non-invasive ventilation, and medications may all contribute to poor sleep in MND. All of these factors can be improved once the main cause of insomnia is identified. Palliative care interventions are useful at any stage of the disease as they improve quality of life and reduce discomfort while keeping individual preferences in mind.

Speech and swallowing

In patients with speech and swallowing difficulties (bulbar impairment), a sore and coated tongue is not uncommon. This is typically caused by the reduced natural movement of the tongue combined with deeper grooves secondary to wasting, which makes it prone to a superficial fungal infection called 'oral candidiasis'. This is important to recognise as it can be effectively treated with anti-fungal medications. Drooling or excessive salivation is a distressing and relatively common symptom of the bulbar form of the disease, which can also be treated efficiently.

Patients with feeding tubes can often continue to enjoy food and drinks in the usual way. Feeding tubes help to maintain weight by delivering sufficient calories, and are often put in place relatively early in the course of the disease. Feeding tubes are concealed under the clothing so they are not visible and they don't impede walking or driving. Feeding tubes are either referred to as RIG (radiologically inserted gastrostomy) or PEG (percutaneous endoscopic gastrostomy) tubes, depending on the mode of insertion. These tubes don't typically interfere with lifestyle, as the dietician can either set up intermittent or continuous overnight feeds depending on individual preferences.

Therapy and research

While the mainstay of MND care is a series of supportive multidisciplinary interventions, the medication riluzole offers survival benefits and is typically very well tolerated. Some nausea and mild gastrointestinal side-effects are sometimes reported, but temporary dose-reduction is often sufficient to improve the symptoms. Another medication called edaravone has been approved in the US but clinical trials in Europe are ongoing to evaluate its therapeutic benefits. A number of other promising clinical trials are under way and recent therapeutic breakthroughs in other neuromuscular conditions, such as spinal muscular atrophy, give cause for optimism for the development of novel drugs in MND.

Research in MND can be categorised into distinct areas, all directly relevant to the development of new therapies. Any research study undertaken in MND is strictly regulated by local ethics committees and international consortia and is governed by European data protection laws. People with MND are asked to provide consent before study participation and are informed how data will be stored, coded and utilised in the future.

The main objectives of research in MND are:

- to develop efficient medications
- gain a better understanding of how the disease spreads

- explore the factors behind the considerable variability in the disease

- develop better diagnostic and monitoring tools.

Genetic studies

Genetic studies focus on the understanding of genetic susceptibility for MND, and deciphering the causes of the disease. While some patients have family members with MND (familial cases), the majority of MND patients are unaware of affected family members (sporadic cases). Genetic studies rely on blood samples from both patients and controls; that is why patients are approached to give a blood sample if they consent to genetic research. The blood is carefully stored and processed, and DNA is extracted in dedicated laboratories. The discovery of novel genetic mutations is an exciting yet labour-intensive process, which often requires large international collaborations.

Epidemiology studies

Epidemiology studies seek to understand gene–environment interactions and the role of lifestyle factors (exercise, sport, smoking, diet), environmental exposures (pollution, radiation) and family history in the pathogenesis of ALS. Data for epidemiology studies are typically collected through carefully designed questionnaires and are either mailed to the patients or administered through semi-structured interviews. The analysis of these data requires considerable care, and complex mathematical models are used either at a population level or in collaboration with other centres. For the accurate recording of disease incidence, potential environmental risks, age of onset, lifestyle and geographical location, national MND registries have been set up to collect, store and analyse data.

Biomarker studies

Biomarker studies seek to identify objective, quantifiable markers to aid early diagnosis, accurate monitoring in pharmacological trials and the development of reliable prognostic indicators. There are two main themes in biomarker research; these are colloquially called 'wet' and 'dry' markers. Research into 'wet' biomarkers focuses on the measurements of various proteins, hormones, markers of inflammation and indicators of cell damage in the blood and spinal fluid. 'Dry' biomarkers focus on the detection and monitoring of MND-associated pathology using non-invasive techniques such as neuroimaging.

Neuroimaging

Specially tuned scanners can generate high-resolution images of the brain and spinal cord and reliably detect brain changes responsible for specific symptoms. This type of research has already helped us to decipher which brain regions are particularly vulnerable in MND and which brain regions remain relatively resilient to the disease.

The large datasets generated by MRI scanners can be analysed to pick up subtle changes over time and help us to understand how the disease spreads from one region to another. MRI studies have shown how the internal wiring of the brain (referred to as the white matter) gets selectively affected and how the cortical part of the brain (grey matter) shows focal degeneration leading to specific disability patterns. Other techniques, such as electroencephalography (EEG) or magnetoencephalography (MEG), can detect electrical oscillations from the brain and characterise the dysfunction of specific neural networks. These studies are also non-invasive and are generally well tolerated by the patients.

Neuropsychology studies

Neuropsychology studies investigate changes in thinking, decision making, memory and language. The characterisation of these changes is important for improved clinical trial designs and compliance with supportive interventions. While neurologists often perform simple screening tests, expert neuropsychologists can detect subtle changes. Neuropsychological tests typically include pen and paper tests and questionnaires, but they can also be administered to patients who have difficulty speaking or writing. Performance on these tests needs to be carefully interpreted using reference values from age-matched controls, therefore no instant feedback is typically given.

Promising international research

Most MND teams are active members of the international MND research community and meet several times a year to exchange information about emerging therapies, new discoveries and breakthrough research findings. Research in

MND has gained unprecedented momentum in recent years; the number of attendees at international meetings has grown exponentially. Awareness of MND has increased considerably thanks to the tireless work of charities, patient advocacy groups and caregivers.

In light of the momentous academic advances and the record number of clinical trials in 2021, the future of MND research looks promising.

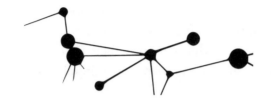

CHAPTER 3

How Will Motor Neurone Disease Affect Me?

BERNIE CORR

The diagnosis of motor neurone disease (MND) has a profound impact on the person who is diagnosed and on that person's family. This chapter is intended to discuss the symptoms of motor neurone disease and the management of those symptoms. There are many useful treatments and interventions, and while currently there is no cure for MND, much can be done to alleviate and minimise the symptoms caused by this condition. This is why the management of MND is focused on symptom relief, promotion of autonomy, crisis avoidance, maintaining independence and enhancing quality of life.

Disease modifying treatment

Currently riluzole (Rilutek) is the only drug licensed for treating MND in Ireland. It is available in tablet and liquid form (Teglutik) and is free with a medical card. Under the drug payment scheme patients only have to pay up to the current maximum of €114 per month. Once they have reached this threshold, any additional costs or prescriptions are free of charge for the rest of that month.

New treatments and clinical trials are being developed and tested all the time. In Ireland, there is a large team of researchers focusing on clinical and translational aspects of MND, and linked with groups all over the world, all of whom are working together to develop new and better treatments for the condition. These researchers are optimistic that new precision-medicine-based approaches towards treatment will help to develop 'the right drug in the right dose, for the right patient at the right time'.

Symptom management of MND

Motor neurone disease is best managed in an MND clinic offering specialised multidisciplinary care. Having multidisciplinary care, or in other words the attention of a number of professionals all working together, is ideal because each profession brings its particular perspective and expertise. People attending a specialist multidisciplinary team (MDT) have access to support from diagnosis onwards, have fewer hospital admissions, increased survival time and improved quality of life. The specialist MDT develops close relationships with community primary care teams, palliative care teams, nursing homes and other hospitals, ensuring a rapid and flexible response to the person's changing needs.

There are many symptoms that may occur following the diagnosis of MND, depending on which part of the body is affected – the arms, the legs, the mouth (bulbar) or the breathing system.

- It is important to understand that MND is an individualised illness and so no two people are the same.

- It is also important to say that not everyone will experience all the symptoms and how one person is affected by the symptoms will differ from another.

- And it must be said that not every symptom experienced will be caused by MND. Something else may also need investigation.

- For this reason we recommend that people talk to their neurologist, GP or specialist nurse about any concerns or worries they might have.

Identifying and discussing the problems and symptoms that may occur can be very frightening. However, it is best to consider everything, to be prepared for all possibilities, so that people can be reassured that, whatever symptoms may develop, there are treatments and interventions that will help the person and their family to cope.

Muscle weakness and cramps

Muscle wasting in motor neurone disease causes weakness. Depending on which nerves are affected, the muscles may become weak and floppy or weak and stiff with painful cramps. The neck muscles can become weak and the head can sometimes fall forward and the chin rest on the chest. This can be extremely uncomfortable and it may affect balance. Again, there are professionals to advise. The occupational therapist and physiotherapist may recommend the use of a collar or neck support. Sitting in a reclining chair with good head support can also help alleviate the discomfort.

If the muscles in the legs become weak, walking may become difficult and a person could be at risk of falls. The physiotherapist may at first recommend using a support in the shoe to help lift the foot and stop it catching on the ground. The occupational therapist may recommend using a lifting and reclining armchair which makes it easy to get out of the chair and into a standing position. If the muscles get weaker, the physiotherapist may advise using a walking stick. If a person has difficulty climbing the stairs, the occupational therapist may recommend a stair lift. If the muscles get even weaker, the occupational therapist may recommend using a wheelchair. For every symptom, there is a recommended intervention.

Understandably, many people are reluctant to use a wheel-chair. It can make them feel as if they are losing their independence, but the opposite is often the case. There are benefits to wheelchair use, as it can actually increase independence, enabling conservation of energy and allowing the person to get out and about more.

Some people may experience weakness in their arms and hands. A weakened grip can make it difficult to pick things up. The occupational therapist and physiotherapist will recommend specialised aids and equipment to help with these kinds of activities of daily living. The physiotherapist will recommend an exercise programme to maintain joint movement, reduce stiffness and discomfort, and maintain strength and flexibility in muscles not affected. Some people may experience pain in the shoulder joint, making it difficult to lift their arm while dressing. Pain can be relieved by taking medication and, if necessary, the shoulder joint can be injected with a local anaesthetic.

If it becomes too difficult to transfer in and out of a chair or bed, the occupational therapist may advise using a hoist. They will help the person and family decide on the most appropriate piece of equipment and provide training to the carer in the use of equipment to make sure that everybody is safe.

Muscles that become stiff (spasticity) due to the illness may develop painful cramps. Taking regular exercise can help. The physiotherapist will be able to demonstrate how to move the limb to ease the stiffness in joints and muscles, and muscle relaxants may also be prescribed.

Staying in the same position

Pain may be experienced as a result of having to stay in the same position for extended periods of time. Being helped to change position may be sufficient to eliminate the pain. A high profile bed with an appropriate mattress may be required to ensure comfort during the night. The occupational therapist may advise using cushions on the chair to help relieve pressure. If it becomes more difficult to move and the pain is causing discomfort, painkillers may be required. Initially pain relief such as paracetamol may be sufficient, and stronger pain relief can be used when necessary. Advice on what is best at any time is always available.

Environmental controls

These are very specific devices that enable people with very little movement to carry out a wide range of everyday tasks around their home. They might include opening and closing doors and curtains, turning on and off the TV or radio, a buzzer for assistance, or using an eye gaze for communication. The appropriate healthcare professional and/or the assistive technology adviser will assess particular needs. The equipment requested is often very specific to the individual person's needs and may take a number of weeks to be ordered and installed. For this reason it is really important to plan in advance to ensure the appropriate equipment is ordered and delivered at the right time to maintain independence and avoid crisis management. Sometimes this is very difficult, as the person has to anticipate that the illness is going to progress and they may feel that by agreeing to get equipment they are giving in to the disease. It is better to think how helpful it will be to have equipment even before it is needed, to practise using it and to know that it is there when/if needed.

Pain

Some people may experience pain, even though the nerves that sense pain are not directly affected by motor neurone disease. The pain may be caused by muscle cramps, stiffness, immobility, skin sensitivity, and stress on joints from muscle weakness and oedema (e.g. swelling of the ankles caused by immobility). The physiotherapist and occupational therapist may advise a passive exercise programme or they may recommend careful positioning to relieve discomfort. If the person is experiencing skin sensitivity, good skin and pressure care is vital; lightweight bed clothing, a pressure-relieving mattress, and cushions may help relieve the symptoms. Simple pain relief may be sufficient. Muscle relaxants may help. However, the best pain relief is the pain relief that is needed, so stronger pain relief such as morphine can also be used when necessary. People are fearful of using morphine and some are worried that it may shorten their life or that they may become addicted, but many people have taken morphine medicines for months, even years, without side-effects.

Fatigue

Fatigue or lack of energy is a common symptom associated with MND. It can range from mild weariness to extreme exhaustion. There are a number of ways of dealing with this and minimising fatigue through management strategies.

- Occupational therapists and physiotherapists know how to advise on energy conservation techniques and labour-saving devices.

- The dietician can advise on good nutrition, and people find it most helpful when they follow that important advice.

- It is also helpful to schedule regular rest periods during the day, and sometimes to use a wheelchair to save energy.

- Adaptations to the environment can make it more accessible, such as using a stair lift to get upstairs or moving the bed downstairs.

- Fatigue related to breathing difficulties should also be discussed with the multidisciplinary team, as respiratory supports may relieve these distressing symptoms.

Always feel free to discuss fatigue with the team. There is good guidance available.

Difficulty swallowing

One of the big fears associated with motor neurone disease is swallowing. The muscles of the mouth and throat may become weaker, so that eating and swallowing may become more difficult. Initially the swallow may feel different, but it may worsen to the point that it becomes difficult to swallow food and drink.

Swallowing should be assessed and reviewed regularly by a speech and language therapist (SALT) in the specialist MND clinic, who will also liaise with a person's community-based SALT. The goal of the speech and language therapist and the dietician is to maintain optimal levels of nutrition and hydration and to reduce choking episodes. The speech and language therapist and the dietician will advise how to modify the consistency of food, making it easier to swallow, and ensure you are getting the appropriate supplements to maintain a balanced diet.

For some people the swallow may become so difficult that they can no longer consume enough food to maintain their normal weight, and gradually eating becomes a very stressful task. Alternative methods of feeding may be considered.

A radiologically inserted gastrostomy (RIG) may be required. A RIG is a procedure to insert a small tube through the skin directly into your stomach. The procedure requires hospital admission. The decision as to whether or not to have a RIG inserted can be a difficult one, so it is important to discuss any concerns with the MDT. The dietician will advise on how to use the RIG and how feeds are given. They will monitor the feeding regime and advise on the amount of feed required according to specific needs. The hospital dietician develops a very close working relationship with the community dietician and public health nurse, providing ongoing advice and support.

Saliva

The salivary glands produce two different types of saliva: thin, watery saliva and thick mucus. The membranes of the respiratory passages also secrete thick mucus, known as phlegm. Everybody produces and swallows about one litre of saliva each day. If swallowing becomes a problem for a person with MND, it may become difficult for them to swallow their saliva, resulting in it dribbling and drooling out of the mouth. This is a very distressing and embarrassing symptom, but, as with every symptom, there are a number of treatment options available.

- Some people like to use a portable suction machine to remove the saliva in their mouth.

- There are a number of medications that may be prescribed to reduce the amount of saliva produced, or a patch can be placed behind the ear, which can be very useful if the swallow is affected.

- Botox injections may be prescribed for patients who have gastrostomy tubes in place.

Some patients may experience thickened mucus in the mouth and throat, which is difficult to clear, or phlegm in the airways, which is difficult to cough up due to weakness in the breathing muscles and an ineffective cough. This mucus may be thick and stringy and cause the airways to become partially blocked. This can be very distressing for patients and their caregivers. Humidification and nebulisers may reduce the thickness and stickiness (viscosity) of the mucus, making it easier to clear. The specialist physiotherapist may recommend using what is called a breath stacker – which helps people who have reduced lung capacity because of muscle weakness – or a cough assist to help clear these secretions.

As with every symptom, it is important for the person with MND to know that there are interventions that can help, so signal if you have distress of any kind with saliva and swallowing.

Choking

Choking is very frightening to witness and to experience. Choking episodes usually occur because of secretions that trickle down the throat due to weakness in the muscles which help us swallow. The specialist team may be able to provide aids such as suction machines, nebulisers and medication that may help relieve the symptoms. The speech and language therapist may suggest different approaches to eating and drinking, in addition to modifications made to the consistency of food and drink. There are a number of things to do to help somebody with MND who is experiencing a choking episode.

1. Try to remain calm.

2. Put the person in an upright position.

3. Open the window to give them more air.

4. If the person has a suction machine or cough assist, use it as advised.

5. If the episode continues and the person is very distressed, get medical advice.

Dry mouth

Some people may experience a dry mouth, which may be caused by the medication they are taking and which can result in reduced fluid intake or breathing through their mouth. The dosage of medication should be checked and changed if necessary. Artificial saliva available in the pharmacy may be helpful. Good oral hygiene is important, to avoid mouth infections. Discuss with the dietician and the speech and language therapist to explore the best ways to increase fluid intake.

Communication

Many people, but not all, may experience difficulty with speech. This is often referred to as dysarthria. Having difficulty with speech has psychological aspects to it. Our speech is an integral part of who we are; as part of communication, it conveys our personality, sense of humour, our views and opinions. Impairment of speech may begin with slurring, hoarseness or a weak voice. Weakness of the respiratory muscles will also affect speech volume, and for some people it may progress to total loss of speech. Difficulties with communication can lead to decreased social interaction and feelings of isolation. Early referral to the speech and language therapist for advice on communication support strategies is advised. The goal is to optimise the communication both for the person with MND and their caregiver.

- Not rushing the person and not interrupting or finishing their sentences may help to create a more relaxed athmosphere.

- It is better not to pretend to understand; this is very frustrating for the person as they can usually tell.

- It is best to check which method the person prefers to use to communicate (e.g. do they prefer to write, or use a tablet, or text on their phone).

• Try to identify key words and have a signal for 'yes' and 'no'.

The speech and language therapist will regularly review the person to ensure assessment and provision of communication aids and training in their use. Augmentative and alternative communication (AAC) devices can be used. Low-tech AAC may include pen and paper, whiteboard and marker, alphabet charts and picture communication aids. The high-tech AAC options may include a voice amplifier, lightwriter, tablet or smartphone, or an eye gaze device. The speech and language therapist will recommend the most appropriate device based on the specific needs of the person.

The speech and language therapist may discuss the possibility of message banking. The idea behind message banking is that the process of recording and then using their messages when needed may help people to feel more in control and keep some sense of identity. If speech quality deteriorates, the person may decide to use an electronic communication device that utilises software with built-in computer-generated voices. This will enable the person's message banking, i.e. the recordings made in his or her own voice, to be used alongside the computer-generated voice. It is important to remember that you do not need speech to have a voice.

Constipation

Problems with the bowel are not usually caused directly by MND, but constipation may occur due to reduced mobility, changes to diet and reduction in fluid intake, and some medications. Constipation can cause discomfort, pain and nausea. Natural changes can be effective. Try increasing your fibre and fluid intake, which may help relieve the symptoms. Laxatives may be used if the natural methods are ineffective, but your doctor or nurse should supervise their use. Diarrhoea can sometimes happen with a severely constipated bowel, so get medical advice if you suspect this is happening.

Other symptoms

As MND is an individualised illness, people may experience a variety of symptoms. Some may experience dry, itchy skin or scalp, which causes discomfort. Others may experience excessive yawning even when they are not tired; this is made worse by the fact that the jaw muscles are weak, resulting in pain and discomfort. Some people may develop a new hypersensitivity to smells, like deodorants or perfumes, or heavily scented food such as curry. As discussed in the chapter in this book by Dr Niall Pender and Dr Marta Pinto-Grau, there can be cognitive and behavioural changes due to degeneration in certain parts of the brain, ranging from mild to significant. There may be problems with attention, planning, memory, word-finding, and general capacity to cope. Behavioural changes can be exceptionally distressing and intervention is crucial when these occur. Uncontrolled laughing or crying or uncontrolled emotional expression may also be experienced by as many as half of those diagnosed with MND. The main message when it comes to symptoms is that if any new or unusual symptoms are experienced, it is important to contact a doctor or nurse, as most symptoms can be relieved.

Breathing difficulties

The thought of having problems breathing is a big cause of anxiety, so it is important to say that it can be helped. Respiratory muscle weakness affects most people with MND. Attendance at the MND specialist clinic ensures regular monitoring and allows breathing muscle weakness to be identified early. As the muscles weaken, less air is drawn into the lungs. This may reduce the amount of oxygen that can be absorbed into the blood. The person may have difficulty exhaling, which then leads to the retention of carbon dioxide (hypercapnia). In this situation, the use of oxygen can lead to further respiratory depression. Oxygen should be used with caution and only following the advice of the specialist MND team. Sleeping tablets are not recommended as they may weaken the respiratory muscles further, making the symptoms worse. Breathlessness can be very distressing but there are interventions that may reduce the symptoms and make the person more comfortable.

The symptoms caused by respiratory weakness may include: disturbed sleep, nightmares, fatigue, headaches, daytime sleepiness, poor concentration, voice becoming faint, weak cough, hallucinations, confusion, difficulty breathing when lying flat, and feeling breathless after mild exertion or even while resting, all of which sounds alarming but help is also available if these occur.

A weak cough will make it difficult to clear the throat, to cough up phlegm and mucus, which may increase the risk of chest infections. Humidification and nebulisers should be considered to help loosen the secretions. Antibiotics may be necessary if there is an infection and, if required, muscle relaxants may be helpful in reducing the feelings of breathlessness.

The specialist physiotherapist can advise on breathing exercises to ensure that the posture is such that it allows for as much expansion of the chest as possible. They may also recommend using breath stacking, a lung volume recruitment bag, or a cough assist, all of which support the ability of the inspiratory and expiratory muscles, which may improve a person's cough and aid secretion clearance.

Non-invasive ventilation (NIV) or non-invasive positive pressure ventilation (NIPPV) refers to a method of providing breathing support to a person by fitting a mask specifically selected to fit your face. The mask will cover the nose and mouth and is connected to a machine that helps support the breathing muscles. NIV has been shown to improve symptoms caused by respiratory weakness, increase quality of life and prolong survival, particularly in people who are compliant in using NIV for over five hours at night during sleep. Some people may have difficulty using NIV, if they have bulbar symptoms, are unable to put on and take off the mask independently, or have cognitive impairment.

Understandably, experiencing breathlessness, struggling to cough, and choking on secretions and phlegm can be very frightening and may cause increased anxiety. Anxiety further affects the breathing and makes the airways tighter, increasing the workload of the respiratory muscles. Anti-anxiety medication can be prescribed to reduce the feelings of anxiety and breathlessness associated with respiratory issues.

In conclusion, for every symptom there is an intervention, so always ask and we will always respond.

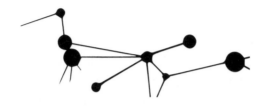

CHAPTER 4

Will Motor Neurone Disease Affect My Mind?

Cognitive and behavioural changes in MND

DR NIALL PENDER AND
DR MARTA PINTO-GRAU

Overview

This chapter is written to explain the thinking and behavioural changes that can occur in motor neurone disease. There are many changes that may occur because of MND and understanding these is important for the person who receives the diagnosis and for the family, friends and carers around that person. Changes in cognition (thinking) and behaviour are due to the changes in how the brain works as a result of MND. The brain controls and manages our daily thinking and behaviour using complex systems that can be disrupted in diseases such as MND. This can result in challenges for MND sufferers and their families.

Thinking and behaviour changes in MND are highly individual. It is important to say that some people with MND will *never* experience changes in how they think and behave, while some may develop mild changes that do not interfere significantly with their ability to complete daily activities and to make informed decisions about their care. For others, however, changes are more significant and can affect their capacity to complete daily tasks and to make decisions, thus requiring their family to make decisions on their behalf. In this chapter we will explain the types of thinking and behaviour changes seen in MND and provide some simple techniques to manage these changes.

How common are thinking and behavioural changes?

Cognitive and behavioural deficits are now recognised as an important feature of MND. Research studies have established that approximately 40 per cent of MND patients present with mild to moderate cognitive and behavioural deficits. Cognitive decline and behavioural change can co-exist in approximately 25 per cent. Up to 15 per cent of patients can also experience what is called frontotemporal dementia (FTD). This is a type of dementia that is characterised by changes in personality, behaviour and language. That being said, not every patient with MND *and* cognitive and/or behavioural decline will experience these symptoms.

What are the most common thinking and behavioural difficulties?

The most common cognitive domain affected in MND is executive function. The term executive function refers to a set of thinking skills such as attention/concentration, planning and organisation, mental flexibility, reasoning and problem solving.

- People who experience executive dysfunction may have difficulty planning and organising tasks.

- They may experience mental rigidity or inflexibility characterised by lowered frustration tolerance, and difficulty with problem-solving.

- Judgement and decision-making may also be affected.

- Language can also be impaired in MND, and often presents in the form of word-finding difficulties so that the person is searching for the word to describe a common object that they know, that is on the tip of the tongue. This is upsetting and frustrating.

- Some people may also show difficulties with spelling, reading or understanding complex commands.

- In more severe cases, individuals can lose the meaning of the words, not being able to recognise them or using them incorrectly in a sentence.

When people with MND present with memory deficits, these are in the form of reduced learning or poor encoding of new information. Moreover, individuals may also have difficulty retrieving information spontaneously.

Behavioural symptoms in MND are quite varied in nature and are caused by MND-related changes in the frontal lobes of the brain. The most prominent behavioural symptom reported in MND is apathy, which is defined as loss of motivation, initiative or interest. Individuals with apathy show passivity and lack of spontaneity. People may need to be prompted to initiate or continue routine activities or previously rewarding activities or hobbies. They may also show reduced interest in starting or sustaining conversation, and show less concern about self-care. Depression or fatigue due to respiratory dysfunction can also interfere with the person's ability to engage in such activities. It is also not surprising that dealing with such a major diagnosis as MND can upset people and make them feel 'What is the point?', so it is useful for families and friends to consider that too when the person seems to be lacking initiative or motivation about things that were important to them previously.

Disinhibition or involuntary lack of verbal and physical self-restraint can also be observed in MND. This behaviour can manifest as loss of manners, socially inappropriate behaviour or difficulties with impulse control. As such, patients can display a general lack of social decorum, such as interrupting others in conversation, failing to wait in line, eating with their mouth open, etc. Individuals can sometimes display inappropriate behaviour towards strangers, such as improper approaching, touching or kissing. More severe behaviours may include poor hygiene, impolite physical behaviours such as flatulence, belching or spitting, or aggressive physical or verbal behaviour. Disinhibited patients may also be more irritable and prone to anger outbursts. Other more severe impulsive behaviours may include reckless driving, gambling, or buying or selling objects without regard of consequences. Of course these are at the extreme and it is important to say that disinhibition is not inevitable but that it happens for some people.

Loss of sympathy or empathy can also be reported in MND, and it is characterised by lack of understanding or indifference to the needs and feelings of others. Family and friends may notice that the person is emotionally detached and distant and this can be difficult for family and close friends to adjust to.

Repetitive or compulsive behaviours may also be present in MND. These behaviours may include simple repetitive movements (tapping, humming, rocking, rubbing, scratching, throat clearing, pursing of lips or lip smacking) or more complex behaviours such as counting, ordering objects, cleaning rituals, collecting, hoarding or walking fixed routes. Some patients can present with altered food preferences and may experience food cravings, particularly of carbohydrates or sweets. Increased or new alcohol consumption and smoking can also be observed.

People with MND may not necessarily be aware of the skills and capacities that they have lost, of all the difficulties and the cognitive and behavioural deficits described above. In the same way, they may not be conscious of the risks associated with physical difficulties, such as falls or choking episodes, and they may also fail to recognise how the demands of their illness can affect their caregivers. It is important then that caregivers understand this and are not hurt by behaviours that are outside the control of the person with MND.

Finally, *emotional lability* is very common in MND, which refers to episodes of spontaneous involuntary crying and/or laughing that can be inappropriate for the social situation. Although these episodes are not associated with an actual experience of the underlying emotion, for example the person may not be finding something funny or sad, the involuntary laughing or crying are uncontainable for people with MND and can be very distressing for them and for those around them.

Why do thinking and behavioural changes occur?

These thinking and behavioural changes emerge when MND affects the connections between two parts of the brain called the frontal lobes and the temporal lobes. These manage our very complex thinking skills like planning, problem-solving, memory and language. When these areas become damaged in MND, the thinking and behavioural skills also become damaged.

How are these changes diagnosed?

The most appropriate method for the identification and diagnosis of cognitive and behavioural changes in MND is a comprehensive neuropsychological assessment. However, due to variations in the presentation of such cognitive and behavioural changes, and the fact that not all patients experience these difficulties, it is recommended that patients are first screened to determine who may need further extensive assessment.

Implications for decision-making

The diagnosis of cognitive and behavioural deficits in MND has important implications for individual patients and their families. These deficits may affect the patient's capacity to make financial and healthcare-related decisions such as acceptance of gastrostomy insertion or the need for non-invasive ventilation. Cognitive and behavioural deficits can mean that the person does not comply with medical advice and treatments, and this can make things more difficult and more risky. Reduced adherence to medical treatments and compliance with multidisciplinary care interventions is problematic. The ability to competently engage in end-of-life decisions can also be affected. Awareness of safety concerns in MND such as avoidance of falls or coping with choking episodes is also an issue in patients with cognitive and behavioural deficits. Some key facts to note are:

- If the person lacks the capacity to make informed decisions, a family member, partner or friend needs to be appointed to make decisions on his/her behalf. Every decision or action taken on behalf of the person with cognitive and behavioural difficulties must be in his/her best interests. You should consult a solicitor to consider the legal aspects of financial and health-related decision-making, as also advised in Chapter 9 in this book.

- Discuss treatment options with the person with MND as soon as possible after diagnosis. It is important that the person feels his/her preferences are validated, and insofar as possible reflect these preferences when making decisions on his/her behalf.

- Allow the person with MND to remain involved in decision-making in some less demanding ways.

Strategies for managing cognitive and behavioural difficulties

- Explain clearly that cognitive and behavioural changes are part of the condition.

- Give a clear structure to the person's day and make it as predictable as possible. Keeping to a routine is very important to ensure that the person can initiate and engage with daily activities.

- Give the patient enough time to make decisions, and offer limited choices and closed-ended questions instead of a confusing variety of options.

- The 'little and often' rule applies. Give the person small amounts of information regularly rather than overload them with too much detail or content.

- Encourage the person to make lists to help organise activities that may need to be done during the day.

- Avoid distractions in order to help with concentration.

- Encourage the person to use calendars, memory aids or phone alarms to help remember appointments or when to take medication.

- Simplify communication to enhance the person's comprehension: speak clearly using simple and straightforward language. Break sentences into short phrases that do not contain too much information.

- Slow down when speaking.

- In people with increased irritability, look for triggers that may prompt bursts of anger, such as tiredness, hunger, thirst or noise, and try to prevent them. In cases of anger outburst, remain calm and avoid arguments. Acknowledge that the person is irritable and angry. It is also important to eliminate environmental stimuli that may be annoying, such as loud noise, or room temperature that is too hot or cold – anything that makes it more difficult for the person to cope.

- Avoid surprises that may create confusion or agitation and keep the environment calm and controlled. If visitors are expected, make sure that the person is aware of this and agreeable. If large gatherings provoke agitation or irritability, avoid them.

A word on caregiver burden

When a loved one receives a diagnosis of MND, there are many changes to expect. These changes not only affect the person with MND, but also the family and people around him/her. Caring for someone with MND can be a very rewarding experience when the appropriate support is available. However, sometimes the caring experience can become challenging. With time, the level of care the person requires increases and caregiving can become very time-consuming. Additionally, apart from caring for a person with MND, caregivers also play a number of other important roles in life and can have many other demands to meet, so trying to keep up with all these roles may also be overwhelming. Moreover, when a loved one receives a diagnosis of MND, it is natural to experience a unique set of emotions which may require time to process and which will influence the experience of caregiving. In this way, caring for someone with MND can sometimes cause physical exhaustion or be emotionally overwhelming. This is known as 'caregiver burden'.

Coping strategies to help you deal with burden

- Take care of yourself – there are times when it will be important to put yourself first, because if you become depleted, exhausted, overburdened or burnt out, you will not be able to care for others.

- Do the practical things such as having a healthy diet and try to get sufficient rest and exercise routinely.

- Take time for yourself. Although it may be difficult to ask for assistance or take time away from caregiving, you need to do that for your own well-being.

- You need practical support. Surround yourself with family and friends who can and will support you and do not be afraid to let them help you.

- Explore the feelings and reactions you may experience when caring for a loved one living with MND. You are living with MND too in a different way, so do think about attending a support group where you can share your concerns and emotions. Some people may also benefit from mental health support (counselling or psychotherapy), which you can access through your GP or multidisciplinary team.

Remember: The better job you do taking care of your own needs, the better job you will do taking care of those around you.

Summary and conclusions

In summary, the cognitive and behavioural changes associated with MND are common and can cause a great deal of distress for the sufferer and their caregivers. These difficulties reflect the effects of changes in the sufferer's brain and are not intentional or deliberate. The person with MND will require careful management and support to cope with these difficulties. Such problems can be challenging for family members and carers too; in some instances they can be more distressing and disruptive than the physical changes associated with the disease. If you or a family member notice these changes, please discuss them with your care team or GP as soon as possible so that suitable supports can be put in place.

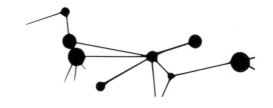

CHAPTER 5

How Will Motor Neurone Disease Affect My Family?

DR MARY RABBITTE AND DR SÍLE CARNEY

Everyone in a family is affected by an MND diagnosis. This chapter will explore some of the common concerns people have when thinking about how MND will impact on their family and friends, their work, their life, their relationships and their social circles. As you learn about the common concerns other people diagnosed with MND have, it may help you feel less alone and to become clearer about what supports you and your family will need.

There are so many questions and emotions that arise the moment a diagnosis is received:

'Is this really so?'

'Could there be a mistake?'

'How will I tell the people I love?'

'How will I tell my friends?'

'Can I keep it from them?'

'Will talking about it be a burden to everyone?'

The questions go around and around because they are big questions that cannot be answered immediately, nor do they all need to be answered at once. Firstly, you have to take the news in, and then you can decide what you want to share with other people, in what way, and at what pace. This chapter will help you start these conversations and give you some tips on how to support yourself and your family when you receive an MND diagnosis.

How do I talk about MND to my family and friends?

After a diagnosis of MND and thinking about how it will affect you, it is normal to start thinking about how this will also change your relationships with your family and friends and how you will talk to people about it.

- Initially it may be easier to discuss your concerns with a healthcare professional.

- You may not feel ready to talk about MND to those that you have close relationships with.

- It may be easier to express your worries, your fears, with someone outside your family and someone who knows and understands how shocking the initial diagnosis often is for people.

- You may not want to talk about it at all. Sometimes people want to go on as if nothing has changed. They think that if they talk about it, it will make it too real.

Whatever you feel or think, it is a normal reaction to the shock, fear and anxiety you have experienced with a diagnosis of MND.

Remember, there is no right or wrong way to approach how you will talk to your own family and friends; it will be your way. However, there may be some things that you can do to support yourself, that may make this easier for you. You may have already included your family or close friends in your discussions with your doctor. If this is not the case, you may want to contact your doctor or another healthcare professional for a follow-up discussion about MND that includes your family or close friends. Always reach out to your healthcare team, as they will endeavour as much as is possible to support you in all aspects of your journey with MND.

Remember, you are in control of when, where and how much you want to tell people about your diagnosis and the impact it has on yourself. Taking charge of this will help you to feel less anxious and fearful. However, although avoiding talking to your family and friends may prevent you from feeling distress in the short term, it may not be a useful coping strategy over time. Despite the wish to protect other people, the support and understanding of your family and friends is important and will improve your quality of life while living with MND. Your friends and family are already likely to suspect something is wrong, and often telling them can be a relief and they can help support you and get support for themselves.

It is important to remember, there may never be a 'right time' to tell people about your diagnosis. It may depend on a number of factors:

- your understanding of the disease and your own reaction to the diagnosis

- your relationship with the person/people you are telling

- how quickly the disease is progressing and the impact it is having on your daily activities

However, it can be really helpful for you to have these conversations as early as possible, so you can offer support to your loved ones, as well as allowing them to provide support for you.

When you and your family have had some time to adjust, you may feel ready to explain what is happening to your wider network of family or friends. It can be a great source of support if you ask a trusted friend or relative to help with this task.

Although having these conversations can be very emotional for everyone involved, telling your loved ones what is happening with clear and simple words can help you and them to avoid misunderstandings in what you are saying.

You don't have to have answers to all the questions

There will be many unanswered questions over the course of the illness, but assure your family that there are services and supports available with whom they can discuss the diagnosis and the illness. They may have questions they do not want to ask you or may want to have a conversation with someone outside the family; these are all totally normal responses. Having open and frank conversations about MND can help your family and friends to feel more included, as well as offering them a space where they can ask questions to get a better understanding of the illness.

Finally, it can be helpful to gently check that people have understood what they were told. When we are in a state of shock, we often do not take in information as easily as expected. By following up with some simple questions you will get a sense of what they have understood from the conversation, but it will also help them feel more relaxed about discussing MND with you in the future.

How do I tell my children?

Family counsellors recommend telling children about serious news as soon as you can and in an age-appropriate way. You may want a close family member or a healthcare professional to be with you when you tell your children, or for them to tell your children for you while you are there. Talking to other parents who have gone through this experience with their children can be helpful. Please remember, if you need assistance in communicating with children and teenagers, the Irish Motor Neurone Disease Association (IMNDA) nurses can support you with this.

Some people may want to 'protect' their children from the illness, but this does not necessarily help your child. Your child will more than likely already know that changes are occurring and may be confused or may even blame themselves. Remember, there is no right or wrong way to tell your children, so it can be helpful to talk through how much and what you are going to say to them with someone you trust. Also, choose a time when you will not be rushed and a location that you and your children can feel familiar with and safe in so that whatever questions your children ask, they can be answered as positively as possible. Answering children's questions as truthfully as possible helps them to feel trusted and secure, knowing that, if they have questions in the future, they will get honesty. Your children will understand that they are loved and included through your reassurance and by you doing positive things with them, such as having regular times for a cuddle and a chat and trying to answer their questions.

The kinds of questions children have are:

- Can I catch it too?

- What will happen to you?

- Will you die?

Remember, try to remain as optimistic as possible, instead of telling your child that you are very sick or dying. You may say something like: 'Well, I am not feeling the best right now, but my doctors say that there are still things we can do.'

Phrasing your responses like this can give hope, without being dishonest. Your child may push certain questions, for example whether someone will die. The best approach at this stage is to be honest but non-specific. It is okay to admit to your child that we will all die at some point, that this is a natural progression of life. It is okay to admit that this is a possibility, but you can assure your child with 'not just yet'.

How to discuss the illness with:

Young children (4 to 8 year olds)

This age group live life substantially in the present, which is not to say that they don't have childhood worries, and when there is illness in a family they are aware of it in their own way. When explaining your illness, try to keep the language simple, and you don't need to go into too much detail about the specifics.

Your child might ask you quite big questions about the illness and seem really upset one minute, and the next they may run outside to play. Being available to listen when they need it is crucial support for them.

Remember, your children won't want or need a lot of information about MND, but they may feel anxious that they have caused the illness or that it may be their fault. Reassure them that they haven't caused the illness and that no one is to blame.

Children at this age can be very preoccupied with germs. Your child may think that MND is related to germs and may be 'contagious', so let them know they can still kiss and hug and that they won't 'catch' anything or hurt you. It can help if you are able to give your partner a hug and a kiss, as this can show your child that it's safe for them to do so too.

However, although we may want nothing more than a cuddle or a kiss from our children, it is better not to put pressure if they are showing any reluctance or fear. It is normal for children to show a natural resistance when someone looks or appears different, but this is usually overcome when it is not made into a big deal. Your child may also need some extra time to adjust to the diagnosis and changes that may be occurring; this is normal, and reassurance and open conversations can help with their understanding of the situation. A useful resource for young children is MND Buddies (see the Other Resources section of this book for further information).

Pre-teens (9 to 12 year olds)

As pre-teens are beginning to want to be included in family conversations, they will want to be respected and listened to within the family unit. At the beginning, they may not want to talk to you about your illness or may not know how to express their feelings, but as they adjust and as things change, they will probably ask more questions. If you are looking to start a conversation with your child, try asking them directly: 'What exactly would you like to know?'

Remember, answer honestly. It is okay if you do not have all the answers, you can let them know that you can ask your doctor at your next appointment. You can also ask them if they would like you to organise a meeting with one of the healthcare professionals on your team to help answer some of their questions; however, let them decide what and how much they want to know.

Teenagers

For teenagers who are already starting to move away from family-centred activities and engage in more peer-related activities related to their age and stage, they may not know how to respond when you tell them. They may present with an adult air and try to protect you by reassuring you that they are okay. They may be juggling their own fears and anxieties and they may not want to burden you with their worry. However, under the surface they may be battling with the fears and emotions that can often come with the diagnosis. Their shock, or their inability to express how they feel, or their wish not to upset you, may make them appear to be unconcerned or callous, while on the inside they will care deeply when you talk to them about your diagnosis.

Because young people are often far more protective of us than we realise, it is important to reassure them that we are able to talk about what has happened. Have regular one-to-one time with them to talk through their fears and anxieties and let them know that you are able to hear their questions and fears. Even when young people do not appear to be listening they usually take in what you say, the way you say it and the love behind it, so don't be afraid to tell them how much you care about the impact on them.

Teenagers and peers

Your teenager may also be thinking about how they will fit into their peer group now, how the illness will change the family dynamic, how they will manage their homework as well as helping around the home, and how much help is enough. They may not want to leave the home for fear they will miss out on time with you, but it is important to encourage them to maintain the support system of being with their friends and continuing their hobbies.

It cannot be said too often that teenagers may not want to talk about how much they are hurting and may be very good at hiding how they are really feeling, so it is vital that you keep communication channels open with them. Teenagers may also be on an emotional rollercoaster with great ups and downs – flattened by grief one day, upbeat and positive the next, then suddenly hostile. Furthermore, they may not want to add to your worries and so may not want to ask you any difficult questions.

It is also normal for teenagers to have feelings of guilt around the illness, as they feel very sad about it, but also they may be resentful that it's made them 'different' from their friends. It is good to acknowledge that they may feel like there is an 'invasion' of their home due to the number of healthcare professionals that may be coming and going, and the fact that the illness now takes up so much of their parents' time and energy. These are all natural and normal responses.

Teenagers, although they are developing a lot themselves at this stage, can see the changes that are occurring due to the progression of the illness, and this may be a source of embarrassment for them. They may become upset if you develop 'emotional lability', laughing and crying unexpectedly or inappropriately, as they may not understand this symptom. Alternatively, if you have other symptoms, such as trouble sitting up straight or unclear speech, they may feel guilt at being embarrassed about what their peers are thinking. This is a normal reaction, and it is important to assure them of this. As one young person expressed it:

'I used to worry about what other people would think when they saw or met Dad in the later stages. I remember feeling embarrassed as the disease progressed and he needed more support, even though everyone told me not to be.'

Spending some quality time with your teenager, engaging in an activity that they enjoy, for example listening to music or going for a hot chocolate, can be a valuable bonding experience for you both. Conversations with teenagers can often emerge during side-by-side activities, for example car journeys, rather than in a face-to-face situation.

How do we cope with what is happening?

One of the best ways to cope is to try to stay in the moment. You can do this by focusing on and prioritising what you can still enjoy with your family and friends, such as spending time with your children or meeting friends for coffee. This more active role can also help you to move out of the shock or sense of numbness you may feel.

There are a number of different coping strategies, some positive, some negative, that people use and it is important to determine which ones are beneficial for you.

There are three common types of coping strategy:

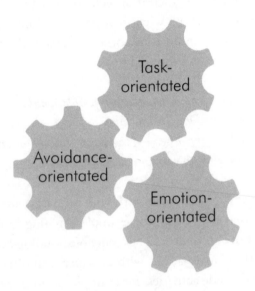

Coping strategies can have long-term benefits or consequences, depending on the situation in which they are used. For example, given the nature of MND, you could adopt an avoidance-orientated coping strategy and deny the diagnosis while focusing on other aspects of life, but in the long term this may prevent you from making important decisions in relation to your future care. Decisions can help you improve your quality of life and make sure you have the type of care that you would wish to have in the future. Caregivers who are avoiding dealing with MND may also be overwhelmed and less able to notice, react and support you or themselves, and because the demands and emotional impact of MND are likely to grow over time, avoidance strategies may be unhelpful for you and your family in the long term.

Adopting a task-orientated strategy can help with the practical jobs that may need to be done, but a purely task-orientated approach can result in avoidance of the impact of the illness. A combination of coping strategies usually offers the best outcomes for the entire family; for example, postponing a particular decision in the short term (avoidance strategy) to allow time to process an emotional reaction and discuss it with others (emotion-orientated strategy), while focusing on day-to-day activities (task-orientated).

The most common piece of advice given by people with MND to someone newly diagnosed is to ask for the support of your healthcare professionals, so that you and your family can make informed decisions in relation to your care. Remember, healthcare professionals such as nurses, occupational therapists, physiotherapists, dieticians and speech and language therapists are available to support you to take practical steps to manage your situation. This can include physical-symptom pain relief and assistive or rehabilitative devices to improve your ability to function.

What if I am depressed?

There may be times when you or members of your family feel depressed or even hopeless. This is a normal reaction to what has happened to you and is not a sign of failure. You do not have to go through feelings of depression and hopelessness alone; you have a right to express these thoughts. This is a life-changing diagnosis, and while there is a lot to remain hopeful for, you have good reason to feel down and low at times. What is most important is that you speak about your feelings, regardless of what they may be, and get support by talking to your family or a counsellor, or your GP, who may decide you need medication to help you through. The IMNDA can support you and your family by providing funding towards counselling sessions.

Healthcare professionals such as your GP will have experience of dealing with people who have thoughts of suicide. Although you may wish to deal with this in the home, it is vital that you seek the support of those who are specifically trained to listen to your feelings in a safe and non-judgemental manner and help you through.

You may also have religious or spiritual concerns, so it may be useful to talk to a chaplain or a trusted spiritual adviser who can help you to maintain a sense of meaning and hope in your life.

Finally, remember that you are a person first, not a diagnosis, in the same way that your family and friends are people with their own lives. Remind people that you want them to see beyond your condition and treat you as a person. There may also be times when you want help with a family issue that is totally unrelated to motor neurone disease.

How can I help my family?

Although you will need the support and understanding of your family and those who are close to you as your condition progresses, your family will also need your support. Be open in communicating your fears and anxieties with your family. You can support your family by speaking up and asking for what you need, either from them or from a healthcare professional. You can also support your family in the following ways:

- Allow them the space to deal with the diagnosis themselves. It is often difficult for loved ones, who can be left with a sense of guilt that it was not them diagnosed with MND, or guilt that they are able to keep doing the things you are no longer able to.

- Provide your family with time and space to express their fears or feelings of anger and frustration; this can bring you closer together as a family by focusing on common priorities.

- Understand their wish, if they want to speak to a healthcare professional about their emotions and feelings. Attending a psychologist or a counsellor can help you and your family to deal with the emotions that arise as a result of the diagnosis and progression of the illness.

- Respect their wishes in relation to the care they are comfortable with providing or perhaps the limits to that care. Although you may not want any professional carers in the home, find out what arrangement suits everyone best and some compromises may become necessary. This is a personal choice and different for everyone.

- It is important to recognise that a decision that is made at one point may change at a later time. It is also important to remember that there is no right or wrong decision, but that what fits to your own personal situation is the 'best' decision.

- Remember how important communication is. Your family will be concerned about you and may feel a sense of frustration in their roles if you do not communicate your needs.

- Finally, try and arrange a time each week where, as a family, you relax with extended family or friends. This can be a safe, loving space where you can fully relax and be yourself.

How will my family be affected and how will family roles change?

Your family may be affected in a number of ways. Younger members may take on greater responsibility such as helping out with household chores. It is important to discuss these changes and how the family roles may change, to set boundaries as early as possible and to allow everyone to say what they are comfortable with. These conversations may need to be had a number of times as things change to ensure that no family members are taking on too much or becoming burnt out. Undoubtedly, this is a very distressing time for people with MND. Family members can experience the burden of caregiving if they are taking on a role they don't feel they are able or ready for. For more intimate tasks like washing and dressing it may be better to receive this care from a professional carer rather than from a daughter or son, and each member of the family will need to recognise their own personal capabilities and limitations. As carers they will also need to provide care for themselves in order to avoid feeling overwhelmed or exhausted.

Signs of exhaustion include:

- chronic tiredness or sleepiness

- headaches

- dizziness

- sore or aching muscles or muscle weakness

- impaired decision-making and judgement

- moodiness, such as irritability.

Caregivers often feel a sense of failure if they are not able to maintain the level of care they once provided, so do encourage your family carers to read Chapter 6 in this book, which gives some tips and strategies to support their own self-care.

What about finances and family role changes?

If you are working outside the home, you may find that as your MND progresses you will not be able to work in the same way as before, which may create a financial strain within the family. Because financial stress can impact the quality of life of a person with MND, do get financial advice and support to cope with any financial changes due to your illness.

There are a number of practical things you can do to support yourself financially:

- Talk to your employer about your condition and seek their support in changing your way of working to help you work for as long as possible outside or within the home.

- Contact Citizens Information to check out all the main services and benefits you are entitled to as a person living with MND. They will be able to signpost you to organisations that you may need to contact as your condition progresses.

- If you have a mortgage and are concerned that you will go into arrears, talk to your bank or financial institution from the start to work out solutions to restructure or delay payments on your mortgage to avoid unnecessary financial pressures. If you are renting and are worried about rent arrears, organisations like Threshold (national housing charity) can provide advice on how to negotiate with your landlord.

- Finally, it is important to contact the Department of Social Protection to find out about your entitlements.

As your condition progresses, it may be necessary for other members of the family to take up the role of primary financial provider. Talk to your family about this as soon as you can if you have to change your role as the primary or sole earner within the household. You may also want to make someone within your family responsible for making financial and care decisions on your behalf as your condition progresses, just in case at any point you lose the capacity to do this for yourself. Chapter 9 in this book on 'Legal Considerations' gives information on getting everything in order, which can take a lot of pressure off you and your family.

Planning ahead is not just practically important but psychologically important too. Whether it is managing your financial concerns or thinking about how to cope in the future, having a plan in place can improve your quality of life and allow you to focus on the important things, including time with your family and friends.

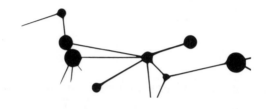

CHAPTER 6

The Caregiver Experience

DR AILÍN O'DEA AND DR SÍLE CARNEY

Introduction

*'My father didn't get a diagnosis of MND,
our whole family did.'*

Caregiver quote

The aim of this chapter is to name some of the important issues for people supporting a loved one with motor neurone disease. We will give you a whistle-stop tour of the research, to flag the kinds of experiences you might expect. We will discuss some issues to be aware of as a caregiver or as a health professional working with MND caregivers, such as risks to physical and mental health. Most importantly, perhaps, we will look at self-care for caregivers.

People with motor neurone disease are both similar and unique. Each person will experience the illness differently and will cope differently. Each family will experience common responses such as grief and worry, as well as coping in their own unique way, due to their individual family situation. Caregiving is not all stress and exhaustion; it can be rewarding and deeply meaningful. Motor neurone disease caregivers also fulfil a very important role in society. The care they provide enables people with MND to remain in their homes for as long as possible, often throughout the illness.

The term 'informal caregiver' refers to family members, loved ones, partners, neighbours – anyone playing a supporting role in the person's life outside of healthcare staff. From the very beginning, when the first symptoms appear, until the end of life, informal caregivers play an enormous role. The impact of MND can be hugely challenging for families. A household may have to adapt, for example, to a situation where the person with MND goes from being the main earner in a home to needing full support with physical care needs. Caregivers often take on a variety of new roles as they support the person with motor neurone disease and the wider family through the experience.

Do I need to call myself a caregiver?

As mentioned at the outset, everyone's experience is unique. For some people supporting a loved one with MND, they do not identify with the term 'caregiver' or 'carer'. You may, for example, be conscious of your relationship with your loved one and not want that to change in a fundamental way; the support you give is simply a natural part of that relationship. The word 'caregiver'/'carer' is used by healthcare professionals and social care services to describe those who provide support to others. While you don't need to call yourself a caregiver, if you do, it's important to know that that does not necessarily change your identity or your relationship to your loved one.

'A stolen future': what the diagnosis can mean for carers and families

A diagnosis of MND means different things for different families. There is no doubt, however, that it transforms the lives of the person with MND and their loved ones. The research has shown that the following kinds of experiences are common for caregivers:

- Shock at diagnosis: feeling profound sadness and grief, feeling the loss of the future you thought was ahead for you and your loved ones, fear about what lies ahead, as well as changes to roles and relationships brought on by MND.

- Coping and adapting: dealing with a moving target as new symptoms emerge and the needs of the person with MND and the family change, coping with new responsibilities and the impact of becoming a caregiver.

- Holding on to what matters: trying to make the most of each day by focusing on living, not dying, holding on to the values that matter to the family and holding on to the identity of the person with MND as much as possible.

Some of these themes may resonate with you, or you may have different experiences. It is important to note, however, that coping for caregivers does not happen in stages or steps. You will be in different states of mind at different times, perhaps going through several different states all in the one day.

> *'Some days all you can do is be kind to yourself. You are doing your best, even if it doesn't feel like enough.'*
>
> Caregiver quote

You may feel, for example, that you have 'dealt' with feelings of loss around the diagnosis and adjusted to it. However, an important change, such as the person with motor neurone disease waking up one morning unable to do something they were able to do the day before, may bring you back into difficult feelings. The graph below illustrates this point.

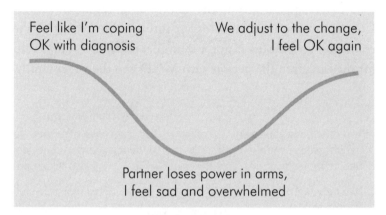

The key thing is to stay open to what supports you may need at different points along the way. An important part of this is allowing yourself, as early as possible, to recognise that you are in a caring role. Many people do not recognise this role unless they are supporting a loved one with physical care needs. Caregivers can be anyone – partners, mothers, children – involved at any level, from helping a person with MND to dress and eat, to giving emotional support over the phone on a difficult day. There is usually a lot to process with MND, long before issues such as possible home adaptations and wheelchairs come into question.

The many aspects of caregiving

'I would say take any help that is offered; take it because you never know until you experience the help how good it could be.'
Caregiver quote

Supporting a loved one through MND is not just about the demands of the illness but includes any number of changes that may happen within the family as a result of MND. Changes to social life and loss of intimacy as a result of the condition progressing can, for example, cause stress and strain for the caregiver, the person with MND and the wider family.

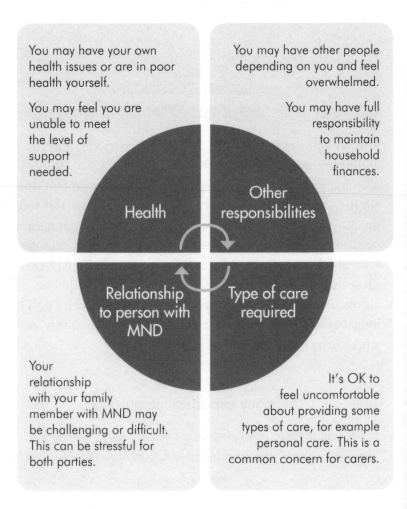

You may have your own health issues or are in poor health yourself.

You may feel you are unable to meet the level of support needed.

You may have other people depending on you and feel overwhelmed.

You may have full responsibility to maintain household finances.

Health

Other responsibilities

Relationship to person with MND

Type of care required

Your relationship with your family member with MND may be challenging or difficult. This can be stressful for both parties.

It's OK to feel uncomfortable about providing some types of care, for example personal care. This is a common concern for carers.

It's worth stopping to consider your own needs too when caring for a loved one with MND. Although your first instinct may be to take on the role without question, taking your own health as well as other factors into account can help you to think ahead, to plan for support, and can improve everyone's experience. Some of the many different aspects of caregiving are outlined in the chart below.

What caregivers have said about their needs

Over the past number of years, a range of studies have been conducted within the motor neurone disease research team based in Trinity College and Beaumont hospital in Dublin. The studies have highlighted the experiences of Irish MND caregivers. One such study was carried out to help our understanding of what kinds of supports are needed. The study found that the need for psychological and peer supports, information and training, and external supports were highlighted most often. The various needs described by caregivers are summarised in the table on the following page.

As shown in the table, the supports needed by caregivers vary and change over time. The right kind of support may not always be available at the right time and this can be a challenge for carers. However, the healthcare professionals on your team and the Irish Motor Neurone Disease Association will always do their utmost to help. They are keen to support you in any way they can, so keep in touch and don't be afraid to ask for help.

NEEDS IDENTIFIED BY IRISH MND CAREGIVERS

1. Practical Supports

- Assistance in applying for home help and carer support.

- Assistance in establishing eligibility and help applying for financial supports.

- Help accessing aids and appliances to help care for their loved one.

2. External Supports

- Caregivers expressed the need for respite, i.e. time away from their caregiving duties.

- Caregivers expressed the need for better communication between healthcare professionals and family caregivers.

3. Information & Training

- Caregivers requested more information and training regarding the diagnosis.

- As the disease progressed, caregivers requested specific care-related training in the form of practical caring tasks (i.e. manual handling, and training for care equipment such as respiratory supports and gastrostomy).

4. Psychological & Peer Support

- Peer-to-peer support: communication with other family caregivers who understand their situation and could provide useful advice.

- Professional support through counselling.

Loneliness and isolation

'Sometimes we don't need advice. We just need to hear we're not the only one.'

Caregiver quote

Taking on the caregiver role can often lead to a sense of isolation and loneliness. You may find it difficult to talk to other family members and friends about the disease. Your loved one may not want others to know they have the diagnosis, which can bring other pressures.

As the disease progresses, the person with MND may become less mobile and it may become difficult for them to leave the house. They may have problems with speech and communication, resulting in difficulty maintaining conversation and expressing their feelings. If you were close, you may feel that you are losing parts of the relationship that meant a great deal. You may even notice changes to their thinking and behaviour. These issues can be especially difficult and distressing for caregivers.

In addition, your ability to engage with your own social contacts may decrease. You may find you have less time for work, leisure, friends and family. Family and friends may not realise the pressures you face, or they may find it difficult to know how to help. This can result in you feeling that you are on your own and no one understands what you are going through. However, it is important to remember that there are services available to support you in your role. There may be no easy solutions to the problems you are facing, but there are certainly people you can talk to who will understand. Often that is enough to get you through.

As treatments improve, people with MND are, thankfully, living longer. This means, however, that more supports may be needed to manage their complex needs over time. It also means that caregivers cannot afford to put self-care on hold. We will look a bit more at self-care and support in the next two sections.

Coping: 'Playing the piano across all the keys'

'Remember, put on your own lifejacket first. Caregivers have to look after themselves. Take it one step at a time. Don't shoulder all the burdens in one day, you don't have to be a martyr.'

Caregiver quote

The research shows that caregivers are at particular risk of experiencing poor health, both emotionally and physically. Believe it or not, sometimes the risk of emotional distress is higher for caregivers than for those for whom they are caring. Part of the reason for this might be that caregivers sometimes feel burdened, not just by the job of caring for the person with MND but by struggling to manage multiple responsibilities, such as caring for other family members and planning ahead for changing needs. So what can you do to mind yourself and protect your health while in a caring role?

Caregiver studies suggest that people use different types of coping strategies. One way of thinking about those different kinds of strategies is to group them into four strands. A caregiver for someone with MND might use the following ways of coping:

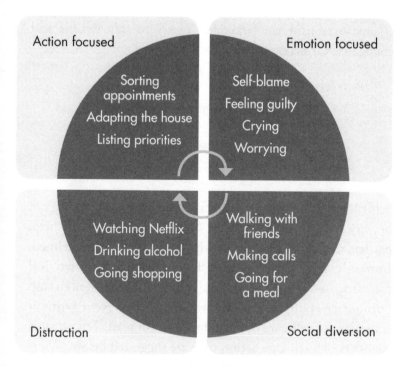

Coping strategies

It is like learning to play the piano across all the keys; it is helpful to be able to use different coping strategies at different times. There are times when social diversion, such as a night out and a drink with friends, might be just what you need. However, drinking alcohol on your own every evening might not be a good idea, for obvious reasons!

Expressing emotions, such as crying and feeling sad, can be an important release valve; however, constant worrying could clearly leave you feeling exhausted. Getting the support of a counsellor or making an action plan might also be a useful response to worry. Finding what coping strategies work for you will be a matter of trial and error. Your needs will also change over time, so remember to try to stay flexible and change tack if necessary.

Making a self-care action plan

'You can't pour from an empty cup.'
Caregiver quote

Self-care is something caregivers often put on hold. It can be very hard to prioritise your own needs and to seek help, particularly at those times when you feel overwhelmed. Ironically, it is when you need help most that you may feel too exhausted to seek it, so try to mind yourself as well to stop burnout creeping in. An important way to prevent burnout is to plan for self-care by making an action plan. Ten possible elements of a self-care action plan are suggested below.

You don't need to take action on all ten points at once. Take even three or four elements and decide how you might fit them into your week. Keep your goals simple and manageable. Change your plans if you find that you are not meeting the goal (e.g. if you can't exercise for half an hour three times a week, try two fifteen-minute walks). Focus on all that you *are* doing and praise yourself when you achieve *any* goals.

TEN THINGS TO INCLUDE IN A SELF-CARE ACTION PLAN

Accepting

If you are supporting a family member with MND, it's natural to feel all sorts of difficult feelings: loss, frustration, fear, exhaustion ... you are having to adjust to an ever-changing condition; accept that you might have a down day or even moments of overwhelming distress.

Try meeting yourself at your own door with compassion, saying, 'This is a moment of suffering. How can I take care of myself in this moment?'

Asking

Don't wait until you're exhausted to ask for help. People around you may be slow to offer help, or the person with MND may be reluctant to bring in outside help, but it's worth persisting. Tell family exactly what you need. Call the IMNDA. Talk to the people on your medical team. The better supported you are, the better you will be able to care for your loved one. Having extra help could make for a more relaxed home environment for all.

Breathing

When we are stressed, we can forget to fully breathe. Imagine that a birthday cake with candles is placed in front of you. You are getting ready to blow out the candles. Inhale deeply and hold for the count of 1, 2, 3, 4. Exhale to blow out the candles to the count of 1, 2, 3, 4. Repeat.

Being

Living in the moment is challenging for most of us. One simple way of connecting with the here and now is by looking around you and noticing five things you can see, four things you can touch, three things you can hear, two things you can smell and one thing you can taste.

Notice when your mind wanders and use the breath or your senses to gently redirect your attention.

Connecting

Take time to connect with people you care about. Connect with the person you are caring for and decide on priorities you want to set together (e.g. quality family time). Take actions that fit with your goals, rather than focusing on outcomes.

Connect with yourself. Keeping a gratitude journal has been shown to nurture a happier mindset. Stop and notice things you are grateful for; it could be as simple as the love of a pet or family member. Creative activity also supports well-being in lots of ways. Start a project, however small. You don't need to be any good at it, you just need to enjoy it.

Eating

It sounds obvious, but busy caregivers can forget to stop and eat. Good food will support your body and mind. Mealtimes can be difficult if you are worried about your loved one coughing or being at risk of choking. Consider taking some meals at a quiet time so you can slow down and taste your food.

Exercising

About half an hour of exercise three times a week is ideal to boost mood. Exercising outdoors and getting light exposure early in the day (15–30 mins) is especially helpful if you notice your mood takes a hit in winter.

Problem-solving

Constant worry can really take from our capacity to enjoy life. Caregivers often have plenty to worry about. Try writing down the problem and brainstorming ideas for how to deal with it. Assess the results of trying one idea and use an alternative if your idea doesn't work. You may also have to accept that the problem can't be solved right now.

Sleeping

Caregivers are often sleep-deprived. Try to keep a regular bedtime routine. Avoid alcohol and caffeine, especially in the evening. Wind down for an hour before bed and avoid bright screens/lights. Keep TVs and phones out of sleep spaces. A cooler room temperature can also help you stay asleep through the night.

Thinking

Overthinking revs up the stress response. When we're feeling down, the mind goes into an unhelpful thinking pattern called rumination. It's 'dog chasing its tail' thinking. It might be the habit of a lifetime, but it is worth stopping and noticing your automatic thinking patterns; catching and redirecting unhelpful thinking will pay dividends (see link to Cognitive Behavioural Psychotherapy Ireland in the 'Other Resources' section at the end of this book).

Unstitching well-worn thinking patterns is not an easy thing to do, however, and you may well need the support of a good counsellor or therapist. Find someone registered and fully qualified. The IMNDA can help cover the cost of this.

Hope is not optimism: living to the end

'It was a privilege to care for my son. I have such precious memories.'

Caregiver quote

The impact of motor neurone disease is undeniable. It can be an extraordinarily tough disease, with devastating consequences for the person diagnosed and their loved ones. Supporting a loved one with MND is not all doom and gloom, however; caregivers and families manage to make the most of what they have, despite the condition. The focus is often on living, not dying, with the goal of enjoying precious time together.

'I had to remind myself that MND was the problem, not my husband.'

'Being a carer doesn't mean that your life ends as well. I still go for my sea swims, that's my escape.'

'Don't feel guilty about taking a day off. It helps everyone in the long run.'

'You need to keep your normality as much as possible. I think that helps the patient as well, so they don't feel a burden. Try and continue life as it was.'

In conclusion, caring for a person with MND can be many things: it can be rewarding and complex, it can be emotional and challenging. MND caregivers deserve huge respect and recognition for the job they do in supporting a loved one living with the condition. In the upset and adjustment that often follows a diagnosis of MND, it is easy to see why caregivers' needs can get lost. This chapter has explored the importance of practical and emotional support for caregivers, as well as describing the importance of good self-care. Caregivers feeling supported in their role is key, as this in turn supports the person with MND and the whole family.

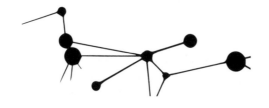

CHAPTER 7

Living with Motor Neurone Disease: A personal account

ANDY MINOGUE

This is me!

I took my first breath in this world on 20 April 1967 in Nenagh hospital, County Tipperary. I have two older sisters and two younger sisters. I spent most of my childhood living in Sallygrove estate in Nenagh town. My childhood was mainly happy as I spent my summers and evenings after school playing soccer in the green area across from our house, as well as just running around. We didn't have much, but we were never hungry and we were always turned out well for communions and confirmations! My mum and dad worked hard to make sure we had 'Sunday best' clothes and they did their utmost to bring us up with good values. I did my Leaving Cert in 1985 at Nenagh CBS. I got very mediocre results, mainly because I was more interested in messing than studying. I had no idea what I would do with my life, but I applied for a temporary position in the civil service and that was the beginning of a thirty-year career. I married Clare O'Brien in 2001. Considering the ambush that lay ahead of me, I could not have married a better woman. We were blessed with two fine, healthy sons. Eoin was born in 2003, followed by James in 2006. As the boys grew up, I would have considered myself a lucky man. Great wife, great sons, good job, great health and no financial worries. At the start of 2015 all seemed rosy. Sure, what could go wrong? Unfortunately, things were already going wrong in my body, but I did not pay much attention to them.

Something is up

It was one Friday afternoon in March 2015 and I was reading emails in my office; all of a sudden I couldn't get a grip on the computer mouse. I tried shaking my arm and hand, but I still could not get a proper grip on the mouse. I was immediately concerned as I knew this was highly unusual. As far as I could see, my arm and hand all looked normal. I could not resist going on to Dr Google. I got plenty of results for arm weakness but only one jumped out at me. It suggested early onset of motor neurone disease. This really grabbed my attention as I was well aware of MND because my sister's boss had passed away from the disease a few years earlier. Two words associated with the disease also jumped off the screen: *progressive* and *fatal*. I spent the weekend very concerned about what may lie ahead. I did manage to grip the mouse the following Monday, but I had started noticing that my whole arm had got weaker.

As I thought more about it, I could recall a time towards the end of 2014 when I had difficulty turning the key in the car door but I wasn't worried at the time. I mentioned it to Clare and she agreed that the only thing to do was make an appointment with my GP. The earliest available appointment was a few weeks away in April but I took that rather than seek an urgent appointment. It was a long few weeks waiting to go to the doctor. I did not help myself by continuing to search Google for more information.

Eventually my GP visit came around. In one way it was ironic that I was attending the doctor about weakness in my arm at a time when I was training for a half-marathon, and that very morning I had completed a ten-mile run. So when the GP asked me how I was I told her about the run, which had gone well, and that, based on that, I hardly needed to be there! I jokingly got up to leave, but then I told her about the issue of the weakness in my right arm. My bloods were all fine but my blood pressure was through the roof because of the stress that I was under. When I was referred to a neurologist I really hoped that she would not utter the letters MND, but quite early in the visit she did. I knew in my heart and soul that she would not suggest this disease unless it was a real possibility.

I knew I was in real trouble and it was at this point that I made an appointment with the employee assistance officer. I broke down crying in front of her as I told her my predicament, and I asked her how I was going to tell a nine-year-old and an eleven-year-old that I was not going to be around for much longer. She tried to reassure me that we were not at that point yet, and to try not to worry until all the tests were completed and results received. I went through a variety of different tests over the next few months including an MRI scan, which did not reveal anything. However, nerve conduction tests did confirm that the signals from my brain were not going all the way to my limbs. Some nerves were dying, which was resulting in muscle weakness. The doctor carrying out the tests said he would send a full report to my neurologist and she would speak to me further. I knew I was definitely going to a very dark place. At this point, I was finding it very hard to sleep and I would often wake up in the middle of the night covered in sweat. I also started to dream about my funeral and I could picture my wife dressed in black with my two boys in black suits. I was terrified to look to the future at all.

Shoe wars!

It was July 2015 and we were in a playground, located in Tralee Town Park. My sons were having the time of their lives, swinging opposite each other on the swings and kicking off their shoes trying to hit each other. They call it 'shoe wars'. I, on the other hand, was living a nightmare. We were in Tralee for a 'lumbar puncture' from my neurologist as part of the ongoing investigations into the muscle wasting in my right arm. If she discovered nothing, the diagnosis could be MND. This thought had me in deep distress and was hanging over me like a black cloud.

When in recent weeks the neurologist mentioned this possibility, all I could see in front of me was the Grim Reaper in his black cloak holding a scythe. I had to work hard to bring myself back to looking at the real person who was sitting in front of me. She was nice, in fairness, but was the purveyor of potentially very bad news! The boys had no idea what I was going through even though the tears were running down my cheeks as I contemplated checking out before they were adults or even teenagers. We had been to the Aqua Dome that afternoon and again they'd had a ball, while I had tried very hard to live in the moment. Now I got up and had a go on the trip wire, if only to stop the crying. I couldn't get them out of the playground and it was nearly dark when I eventually dragged them away.

Back at the hotel I went down to the bar for a pint. This was not the normal relaxing drink that I would have when staying in a hotel. This was simply a sleeping tool, as I knew that I would get no sleep without a drink. I followed it with two more and did fall asleep as a result. I was up before 7 a.m. the next morning, so I decided that I would walk to the hospital rather than drag the boys up. I sobbed all the way to the hospital, and as the journey took twenty minutes, it is fair to say that my reservoir of tears was well depleted! I had to regain my composure at the hospital because there was a big crowd in the waiting room. No doubt some folk could see the black under my eyes.

Coping mechanisms

Getting a diagnosis of MND is devastating! It is like being hit by a bus. Even though I knew it was coming, it still shakes you to the core. Another emotion that I remember having was one of pure deflation. All of the hopes and prayers that it would be any other condition were well and truly demolished! I was going around in a daze for the rest of that fateful day and for some time after. While I tried to register what was happening and tried to find a way to move on, I knew it was in what would be a very different life.

I did eventually move on, and even though it took me about two years after diagnosis, acceptance of the situation was a big factor in enabling me to do so. I was of course making many adjustments during those two years but emotionally I still had not fully accepted it. I would input my symptoms into Google and try to find other conditions that matched them. For instance, for a certain period I hoped that I had multiple sclerosis (MS). When I put this to the neurologist, she told me that with MS you do not have muscle wasting and that is the main difference. She also dismissed any other conditions that I put to her, but in a nice way. I felt that I had to tick those boxes anyway. After I finally accepted the condition I felt I could move on with my life. Even though I was now physically worse off, I was mentally in a much better place. My attitude was, 'It is not a good situation but it could be a lot worse, and let us make the best of it.'

So how do you actually cope when you are living with MND?

I decided that what I would do is do everything that I can do for as long as I can possibly do it. I was lucky in that I have a rare type of MND called flail arm syndrome. I received this upgraded diagnosis in November 2016 and it was as welcome as it was surprising! This is a less aggressive type, with a better prognosis. Accordingly, the changes that I was encountering were all gradual, so I have found myself making incremental changes over the last six years or so. The list of things that I have given up over that time is very long, but I prefer to think about what I *can* do rather than what I cannot.

Leaving work in April 2016 was a massive change. After thirty years of working full time, I had enough of trying to write with my left hand, and failing miserably, as well as struggling to type and use the computer mouse. I found myself having difficulty passing the days. My main activities were school runs, running and reading. Eventually I learned to adjust to the new regime. I definitely found that keeping busy, particularly keeping my mind busy, was very important for dealing with this situation. I also found it very useful to find other ways of doing things by making ongoing adjustments. For instance to keep running, a pastime that was more of a love than a hobby for me; I designed my own slings to wear across my arms to stop the flailing as I ran. That enabled me to stay active right up until October 2018. This I found excellent for my mental well-being. I bought a new, specially adapted car and, even though I only ended up getting six months out of it, it was six months of driving that I would not have got otherwise.

Around the house there are many things you can do, such as getting an electric toothbrush, kindle, electric shaver and various other gadgets that can help you when you have no power in your arms and hands. Another big factor in coping is simply asking for help. I am very lucky to have Clare and two sons to help me. At this stage, I get up at 8 a.m. every weekday and I do twenty minutes on the exercise bike. Although my balance is very poor, I can still walk into the shower, but I do require assistance with drying and dressing. I don't need too much attention for the rest of the day, with the exception of help with eating.

Another thing that helps me to cope is that I get to spend more time with my two sons. Six years ago I was convinced that I would be dead and buried by now. I am happy to be alive, although I lost my voice during 2020. From the time I left work in April 2016 I have been here with my sons for all their summer holidays, mid-term breaks, Christmas holidays and Easter holidays, and any time they are off school. This is something I would have missed out on had I still been at work. Therefore, this is without doubt a real positive that I have taken out of a very difficult situation.

Sometimes you have to laugh!

There is nothing funny about living with MND; however, I think that having a sense of humour can help make the journey a bit easier. In fact, you could argue that having a sense of humour is even more important at times like this. I was paid a big compliment in 2018 after I told two good men that I had MND. We had just consumed a few beers and one of them said, 'Well you're still good craic anyway!' In recent times, people have said nice things to me, for example that I am inspirational and very brave, but being told I was still good craic meant even more. I have not been very sociable over the last few years and there are many people I would have seen regularly that I have not seen for a good long while. While I have not been to the pub of late, my friends still call to watch matches and we have the craic.

In the course of my journey, I have found a few highs with the lows. Sometimes the glass is definitely half-full. For example, I am bald. When I was in my twenties this was something that used to bother me. Now, however, every time I walk into the shower I am glad that I do not have hair as I cannot lift up my arms to wash it.

I was in A&E with a minor issue in June 2020 and a nurse asked me if I had any other conditions apart from MND and I burst out laughing. She was confused, and when I regained my composure I said, 'Is MND not enough for you?' Then she laughed! I find that if you don't laugh you might cry, and everybody knows that laughing is more enjoyable.

Over time, I have developed a mantra. The words *battle hard* spell out how I have coped over these difficult past few years. I hope these words can help others as they have helped me.

B is for busy. Keep yourself occupied in some way or other, particularly if you have had to leave work.

A is for acceptance. Once you accept the illness, you can move on.

T is for targets. Give yourself something to complete or achieve.

T is for treats. Treat yourself – don't wait for others to do it.

L is for letting go. Let go of what you can no longer do, but do not look back in anger.

E is for exercise. Do whatever you can do, for as long as you can.

H is for headspace. Get your head right in order to face this battle; seek professional advice.

A is for adjustment. Make adjustments which make your life easier and less stressful.

R is for rest. Take time out for a lie-down every afternoon or evening – you will need it!

D is for diet. A good nutritional diet is important for keeping your strength up.

I hope that telling my story will help others who are on this journey or who may have to face it in the future. It is love that sustains us through it, and nothing reflects that love more than the care of our families when the chips are down.

Andy died in July 2021 leaving a legacy of his words for others as he wished to do. Ar dheis Dé go raibh a anam.

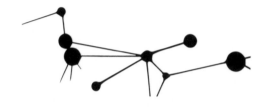

CHAPTER 8

Facing the Future: What to expect from palliative care

MARGARET WINTERS

Introduction

The aim of this chapter is to give an overview of the support that the palliative care team can provide when someone receives a diagnosis of motor neurone disease (MND). Living with a condition such as MND can be challenging and frightening, not only for the person with the diagnosis but also for the person's family members, friends and carers. Everyone needs support in this context and support is available for everyone who needs it. A major source of support is palliative care.

What is palliative care and how can it help you?

Palliative care is concerned with quality of life from the point of diagnosis to the time of death. It may be thought of as an additional layer of support for you and your family in living with and coping with your illness. Involvement of the palliative care team does not automatically mean that you are going to be admitted to a hospice or that you are dying. Palliative care is designed to help you receive the best possible practical and emotional support so that, as your symptoms present and progress, you not only have the support of your GP and primary care team, but also the palliative care team.

You can receive palliative care at home, in hospital, in a nursing home or at a hospice. There are thirteen hospices in Ireland, currently with a total bed capacity of 258 beds. This is complemented by a community palliative care team in each county in the Republic of Ireland. Some hospices also provide hospice day services and outpatient services.

Referral to palliative care

Referral for palliative care does not mean that you have reached the end of your life, it just means being prepared for what lies ahead, even years ahead. Many people are fearful that palliative care or hospice care means they have reached the final stages of a life-shortening condition. It does not mean this. While people are referred to the palliative care service at different stages of their illness, consultants and GPs are advised, once a diagnosis of MND is made, to refer people as soon as possible so as to maximise the support provided to the person with MND and the family.

In the past, referral for palliative care was usually made at the end of life, but things are different now and research has shown that both patients and families who are referred to palliative care benefit enormously from their services and support. Palliative care not only encompasses end-of-life care but also focuses on living and quality of life.

If you need to be referred for palliative care, the Health Service Executive (HSE) in Ireland has made a referral form available for ease of referral, which can be completed by your GP or referring consultant. It is important to remember that your own GP remains your primary carer after referral to the palliative care team, and the palliative care team should be seen as an additional layer of support for patients and their families.

The role of palliative care is to manage symptoms, identify and plan future care needs, guide you through changes, and provide a wide range of supports to you, your family and those who care for you. The palliative care team works in partnership with:

- your hospital team
- public health nurse
- physiotherapist
- occupational therapist
- speech and language therapist
- any other community support services which may be in place in supporting you.

Palliative care may be delivered by a multidisciplinary team in a variety of settings, including hospital, in your home, hospice day or outpatient service, or in a hospice. When the referral is made, you may be seen by the team either in the hospital (which is the hospital palliative care team) or at home (the community palliative care team). Either way, you will be met by a doctor or nurse who will assess your condition and your needs. They will talk to you about any concerns you have and make a plan with you to manage your illness and support you and your family so that your individual needs are understood and met. To support you they might need to refer you to other members of the team, depending on what you need. The palliative care team will link with you on a regular basis to review your symptoms and manage any changes.

How can the palliative care team help you?

The palliative care team is available for you at every stage of your journey through MND. All team members are equipped with specialist knowledge and skills in supporting people with life-limiting conditions and their families. The team members may vary depending on where you live but include doctors, nurses, physiotherapists, occupational therapists, complementary therapists, social workers, chaplains, pharmacists, speech and language therapists and dieticians. Volunteers also form an important part of the team and, like other team members, they have received special education and training in palliative care.

As each person's experience of MND is individual to them, the aim of the palliative care team is to provide ongoing assessment of your condition, managing symptoms, providing physical and psychosocial care to you, and support to your family and caregivers. While each team member brings their own set of knowledge and skills to the caring situation, the combination of all the team members ultimately makes the difference in your overall management.

Psychosocial care

Psychosocial care refers to social, emotional and spiritual care, not only for the person with a diagnosis of MND but also for their family members and caregivers. As MND progresses, you may experience a number of losses over the course of your illness. These losses can be both physical and psychosocial, may vary from one person to another, and may have differing degrees of impact on you, your family and caregivers; for example, not being able to work, play sport or drive, or, as the illness progresses, a change in intimacy or needing help with washing, dressing and moving.

You may have experienced an array of symptoms for some time before diagnosis. These symptoms can often include personality changes, which can potentially create tensions or distance in relationships. When the diagnosis then comes, people can begin to review the previous changes in a new light, but still have to deal with the impact of those changes on their relationship. Many people with MND and family members describe this as the beginning of the losses they experience as the illness presents. Many will also have dealt with delayed diagnosis, or misdiagnosis en route to the diagnosis of MND. This can create confusion, upset and anger and can require support to process. Such experiences call for skilled psychosocial care and interventions to support the person with MND, their families and their caregivers. The palliative care nurse and social worker can provide this support to you and/or your family members.

A diagnosis of MND may bring up a number of feelings, including shock, anger, disbelief, fear and sorrow. You may have questions such as:

- Why me?

- Why now?

- What is going to happen to me?

You may begin to review your life, try to make sense of your situation and wonder what it is all about. You may be faced with various challenges and struggles as you adapt to your diagnosis.

This is where the notion of us being spiritual beings often comes into play. Spirituality affords people an opportunity to reflect on what gives life meaning. Facing serious illness may raise many questions about our values and beliefs. All members of the palliative care team provide spiritual care, while chaplaincy support is available if required.

Changes to roles and relationships

Roles and relationships within the family change with MND. A spouse may become a caregiver or the main earner may become a patient. This can bring challenges and adjustments, including physical, psychological and financial, for the person with the diagnosis and the family. There may be little time for fun or intimacy as the home becomes busier with healthcare professionals calling, appointments, and frequent trips to the GP or pharmacy, as well as the usual everyday living activities such as getting the children to school or managing a household. Allow friends and family to help. Give them practical tasks when they ask if there is anything they can do.

As already outlined in this book, young children in the family are not immune to the changes that are occurring in the family environment. They may not know exactly what is happening but they are sensitive to a change in atmosphere and emotions within the family. There is a natural instinct to protect them from worries or distress, but it can be helpful to talk as openly as possible to them, at a level and pace appropriate to their age. This is important because sometimes what children imagine can be very confused, and they may keep their worries or fears to themselves. Once again, the palliative care team can support you with this.

Allow children to help at a level they are comfortable with, as being useful can help them to feel involved and valuable.

This may be generally helping around the house rather than with medical care specifically, but whatever their input, it keeps them connected and helps them too.

A teenager may be comfortable in helping with practical tasks, such as cutting the grass and putting out the bins, whereas a younger child may be happy to sit cuddled up with you to enjoy their favourite television programme.

It is important to remember that, even though you may no longer be able to physically participate in the same way in some family activities, or that adjustments are needed to maintain intimacy, you are still the same person. Your diagnosis does not define you. It is about finding new ways of continuing to participate in family life. The palliative care team can sensitively discuss these changes with you and offer practical suggestions.

In recent years we have come to understand that MND can be accompanied by cognitive changes. What this means is that you may experience changes in the way you think or behave, or your reasoning may change. Some people find they have mood swings, loss of inhibition, a lack of empathy or reduced reasoning, and problem-solving may be difficult too. For many people, these changes can be subtle, while for others they may be more pronounced. Sometimes people may experience uncontrollable emotions such as inappropriate laughter or crying, so it is important for you, for family members and for carers to be aware of this possibility and understand that it is part of the condition.

All families have a past, a present and a future. Families are complex systems that change over time. Following a diagnosis of MND, pressures are exerted on the present and on the future. Struggling to adapt to a family member being diagnosed with

MND and witnessing the decline in their condition can cause disruptions in family dynamics, as all parties enter uncharted territory. In terms of family relationships, this can result in family members either moving closer together or moving away from each other.

Families may struggle with the unpredictability and un-certainty of the illness. Discussions around prognosis can be difficult. Making sense of this and considering the impact for future care planning can be important. The palliative care team can support you and your family with these conversations at an appropriate pace, helping you to manage the information you have received about your illness, the symptoms and the prognosis, and to consider how best to address the future.

- Meeting with a palliative care social worker as an individual or as a family benefits both the person with MND and their family.

- It provides a safe therapeutic space to react, express and make sense of this illness, with a professional who has therapeutic skills and practical knowledge to impart.

- This enables people to share information about the illness and to discuss what it might entail in terms of the age of family members and their ability to adapt to the new situation.

- It can offer support in understanding and living with MND in the family.

All these supports are designed to help the person with MND and the family to cope as they experience the stress of the ongoing process of change and adjustment that living with MND entails.

Planning ahead

Advanced care planning is a major part of palliative care. Before speech and communication become challenging, it is important to consider your future wishes, plan ahead and make these plans known to your family and care team.

A diagnosis of a serious illness may raise issues you have never had to consider before. If planning ahead is too daunting or overwhelming, you don't have to look at everything at once. Some people prefer not to think about this at all, while others prepare for the later stages of MND as soon as they can.

Some things you might wish to consider include:

- If I become less well, how will I manage?

- What support is there for me and my family?

- Who will look after me?

- Who do I contact if I am unwell?

- Is it feasible to stay at home as things change?

If you need more practical help at home, the palliative care nurse can liaise with your local public health nurse (PHN) about accessing additional care supports available in your area.

It is also not unusual for some people with MND to think about dying and how it may happen, whereas others may find it very difficult to consider or discuss. It can be helpful, however, to let family or friends know your wishes so they can do their best to carry them out. If it feels too difficult for you to start these conversations, the palliative care team can support you with this.

Other areas that need consideration include what you do *not* want to happen, such as being resuscitated if your heart stops, or transferred to hospital if treatment would not be beneficial, while decisions may also need to be made around the insertion of a feeding tube, assistance with breathing via a ventilator (breathing machine), and the treatment of recurrent chest infections. There may be practical issues to consider too, such as making a will or letting someone know your computer passwords or financial details if you are unable to access or manage these things yourself.

As your condition changes, the palliative care nurse will review you more frequently to manage any symptoms and offer support. It may be helpful to have some medications available at home in case other symptoms arise. If you are unable to swallow medication, an alternative method such as a subcutaneous infusion or syringe driver may be used. The palliative care nurse will work closely with your GP and care team to ensure you are as comfortable and well supported as possible.

Sharing your preferences and concerns with your primary care and palliative care teams is helpful in planning your care. It can also help to reduce concern for you and your family, so that you can focus on the things you really want to do.

Your experience of MND is unique to you and your family and there is no script for it. What is right for you may not work for someone else, but know that the palliative care team will guide and support you through everything you need, at your own pace. Conversations about the future can be difficult, especially if a crisis occurs, so if you can, it is helpful to explore these issues in advance and have a plan in place at an early stage in your illness. Members of the palliative and primary care teams can sensitively have these conversations with you and your family. This may provide some reassurance, knowing that things have been discussed and a plan is in place.

We may all think about our own death from time to time or have an idea as to what we would like to happen after our death in terms of a funeral or remembrance service.

You might consider discussing your wishes with your family while still able to, as this might allay any anxiety they may have about funeral arrangements. You may also consider making contact with a local funeral director, again to discuss your wishes, and also perhaps the costs involved.

Engaging in such conversations can afford family members a final opportunity to fulfil their loved one's wishes, which can also help in the grieving process.

Bereavement support

Death comes to all of us in time. However, medical conditions make us much more conscious of our mortality and much clearer about making arrangements for those we love and leave behind. People naturally worry about how their family will cope when they are gone, but be reassured that a significant aspect of palliative care is bereavement support for your family after your death. It may be reassuring for you and your family to know that support is available, as even considering the possibility of a time in the future when you are no longer with them can be overwhelming for everyone.

Grief may be described as the price we pay for having loved someone. It is something we all experience, yet no two people grieve in the same way, not even in a family. We all have a different relationship with the person and we all have different personalities, therefore how we cope and grieve will be unique to each of us.

Sometimes it can help to talk to someone outside of your family and friends. The palliative care nurse will continue to support your family and if necessary offer extra support through the social work service. The palliative care social worker is trained to understand the many aspects of grief and bereavement and can accompany your family on their journey through grief.

Conclusion

Palliative care is an approach to care which looks at the whole person and their family, not just their diagnosis. I hope that this chapter has taken some of the fear away from a referral to a palliative care service. It has outlined the process/journey from referral, managing potential symptoms, coping with change, practical issues to consider when thinking ahead, to ongoing support for your family.

Your illness does not define you, and with the help of a range of healthcare professionals, we will support and care for you every step of the way.

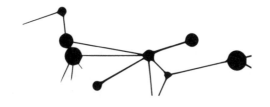

CHAPTER 9

Legal Considerations: Information on wills and managing your assets

ANNE CORRIGAN

When a person receives a diagnosis of a serious medical condition, it is important to take some time to come to terms with that news. Often, soon afterwards, thoughts can turn to various things that the person wants to organise. Usually close to the top of the list is thinking about how to arrange financial affairs, including making a will if one is not already in place, or reviewing an existing one. Many people are also aware that it is possible to make an enduring power of attorney, or 'living will' as it is sometimes called, and that is something they often want to investigate.

This chapter gives information on the most common issues you might want to address, and we hope that it will give you sufficient information to help you make choices. Of course, everyone's financial and family circumstances are different. Some people are part of a family where all of the family members are independent adults, while others have minor children or vulnerable family members. Here we can only give you general information, and you should always seek your own independent legal advice.

General and enduring powers of attorney

There are two types of power of attorney that you might find helpful.

General power of attorney

A general power of attorney is a short document you can sign to authorise one or more people (known as attorneys) to act on your behalf. The attorney can be a family member or anyone else you choose, such as a friend or professional adviser.

Usually the attorney is given the authority to do anything on your behalf that you could do yourself. It is also possible to sign a more limited form, which would restrict the attorney to only doing specific things listed in the document. General powers of attorney are usually used for administrative convenience, to delegate tasks to the attorneys you have appointed. You still retain full power to act personally instead if you wish. Naturally, when giving someone authority to deal with your financial affairs, including for example the authority to make debits from your bank account, it is important that the attorneys chosen are of the utmost integrity.

A general power of attorney ceases to be valid if you become mentally incapacitated. If you want to appoint attorneys who could manage your affairs in that event, it is necessary to sign a separate document known as an enduring power of attorney, described below. Both general and enduring powers of attorney cease on your death. The executors you have appointed in your will then become responsible for dealing with your assets. If you owned assets but died without making a will (intestate), your estate would be dealt with by administrators appointed by the High Court Probate Office, as covered later.

Enduring power of attorney or 'living will'

You can appoint one or more attorneys to act on your behalf in the event that you become mentally incapacitated by signing a document called an enduring power of attorney (EPA). This would not come into effect unless you became mentally incapacitated, and so the EPA might never be required at all. However, should you become mentally incapable, then your attorneys can be authorised to take responsibility for your financial affairs, as well as taking certain personal care decisions on your behalf. This ensures that the people you have chosen will be those exercising power over your finances and making decisions on your behalf. If you became mentally incapable without an EPA, your family or next of kin do not have legal authority to deal with your assets. If it became necessary to do so, they would have to apply to make you a ward of court. This is more complicated and expensive than making an EPA. The High Court will appoint a committee (which may comprise members of your family) to look after your interests, and it will take control of your financial affairs.

Because an EPA has the advantage that you can select the people you think most suitable to take care of your affairs and well-being, you may wish to make an EPA as an 'insurance policy' so that it can be used if required. It is important to understand that you can only make an EPA when you have mental capacity to understand the nature of the document. Therefore, if you think that you would like to put one in place, you should take action sooner rather than later.

The regulations on EPAs require them to be in a standard format. You can specify one or more persons to act jointly (i.e. they must act together) or jointly and severally (i.e. they can act together but each of them can also act independently of the other). As you are entrusting your assets to other people, it would be prudent to appoint at least two attorneys, but you may feel comfortable giving your spouse, life partner or some other trusted person sole power over your affairs. You can also nominate alternative attorneys to act in the event that your first choice attorney(s) is/are not available for any reason. You can specify how much authority you are giving to the attorneys. These powers can be extremely broad to extend to all of your property, or you can place limits on their authority. You can also give your attorneys power to take personal care decisions on your behalf, such as where you should live and who you should see.

The attorneys are permitted to apply your money and assets for your benefit. They may also use them to benefit other people by doing what you might be expected to do to provide for their needs; for example, if you have a spouse, partner or minor children who are financially dependent on you, your attorneys can provide funds for their maintenance in the same manner as you had been doing. The attorneys may not use your money or property to make gifts unless you have specifically authorised them to do so. Even if you have given specific authority, the attorneys can only provide gifts in limited circumstances to persons related to or connected with you, to mark an occasion such as birthday or marriage anniversaries, or to charities which you had or might be expected to support. The amounts of any such gifts are subject to any restrictions in the EPA and have to be reasonable in the context of your assets.

At present, it is regarded as doubtful that an advance healthcare directive can be included in an EPA. An advance healthcare directive gives directions on the type of medical treatment you would want if you were not able to decide on such treatment at the relevant time the need for it arose. It is generally considered that the regulations governing EPAs do not permit the delegation of power to an attorney to take decisions on the medical care of another person. However, despite this doubt, some people opt to include an advance healthcare directive as they consider it to be an important expression of their wishes. Depending on what has been written, the directive could be construed as the giving or withholding of consent to certain types of medical treatment, and so could be regarded as enforceable on that basis, but at the present time uncertainty still surrounds advance care directives and it may be several years before that changes.

There are significant safeguards surrounding the making of an EPA and it is advised that anyone considering making an EPA gets professional advice, as there are so many formalities in setting one up. It is important that every step is carried out carefully with your full knowledge, understanding and consent and with checks and balances to protect you.

Making a will

Why should you make a will?

Everyone should make a will and, over a lifetime, many changes may be made to ensure that what you wish is carried out. A will is also important because any power of attorney, whether general or enduring, ceases to have legal effect on a death.

Legal formalities of making a will

You must observe certain legal formalities when making a will, as follows:

- It must be in writing.

- It must be signed by you or by some person instructed by you.

- The signature must be made or acknowledged in the presence of two or more witnesses present at the same time, who must also sign the will.

- You must have attained the age of eighteen years or must have been married.

- You must be of sound disposing mind at the time you make your will.

The witnesses to your will should both be independent, i.e. neither the witness nor the spouse/civil partner of the witness should be beneficiaries under the will. Otherwise, while your will is regarded as valid, any bequest to the witness or spouse/civil partner of the witness will be null and void.

Executors and trustees

One of the most important decisions you have to make when making a will is choosing who the executors and trustees will be. As with powers of attorney, apart from the case of a spouse or life partner, it is usually best to appoint a minimum of two people.

To explain the difference between the roles, the duty of the executor of an estate is to identify all of the deceased's assets and bring them under control; to pay funeral costs, costs of dealing with the estate and any debts had, and then pay what is left to the persons entitled to it under the terms of the will. If the people who are entitled to the residue are all adults who take specific shares outright, the job of the executor is complete after that distribution has been made. However, sometimes it is not possible to bequeath a legacy or share of an estate to a beneficiary outright because he or she may be a young child, a person with a disability, or otherwise vulnerable. In that case, the legacy or share of the estate is entrusted to a person known as a trustee, with instructions that the trustee is to apply the bequest for the benefit of the beneficiary in question. It is possible, and very common, for the same people to be named as both executors and trustees.

It is important that those selected to be executors and/or trustees of your will are people of the utmost integrity. You should have confidence that your executors will promptly and properly deal with all of the administration and management work arising out of your estate and that the trustees will manage any trust established under your will. If the will has established a trust for minor children or other vulnerable beneficiaries, it could be in existence for several years. It may require significant time and attention and you must be satisfied that the trustees you select will give it that time and attention, or will obtain professional assistance to ensure that it is properly managed.

It is also important to consider possible conflicts of interest. It can cause problems if the executors or trustees who are appointed have financial or other interests that are in conflict with the interests of the beneficiaries.

Guardians of minor children

A parent may appoint a person to act as guardian to minor children, either by deed or by will, until they reach eighteen years. Generally, in the case of a married couple or civil partners a guardian is only required to act in the event of the death of the last survivor of the parents.

The guardians appointed should be the people who the parent believes would provide the children with a warm, loving home. The choice of guardian requires a great deal of thought. Luckily for most people obvious candidates spring to mind.

Where possible the parent will wish their children to remain close to their existing home and school, and those are factors to be taken into account in selecting the guardian. It is possible to leave a detailed letter of wishes for the guardians, setting out the parent's thoughts on issues such as the education, welfare and general upbringing of the child.

The person or persons named as guardians can also act as executors and trustees of the will. However, often different people are chosen for these roles, in the belief that they can bring a different mix of skills to the table. A testator (someone who has made a will) might prefer that the person who is providing a home and acting as guardian to the child does not also have to deal with the responsibility of financial management of the estate, and allocation of funds for the child's living and education expenses.

When should you consider including trust provisions?

A range of circumstances can arise as a result of which you may consider establishing trust provisions in your will. Establishing trust provisions in your will is likely to be because you think that one or more beneficiaries would not be able to effectively manage the inheritance you leave to them. In such a case, you can safeguard their interests by arranging for people you trust to manage their inheritance on their behalf.

Trusts for minor children

If you have minor children, you will be giving a great deal of thought to the type of financial provision you want to make for them in your will. If you are married or in a stable partnership, you may wish to structure your will so that the bulk or all of your estate passes to your spouse or partner. On the death of the survivor of you, the estate will pass to your children. That can be a very good model, but it might not be suitable in every case, for example if your spouse or partner had any vulnerability that might put the inheritance at risk. Again, your solicitor's advice on the best way to manage different circumstances is advised.

If you are single, widowed, separated or divorced, then making provision for your children is likely to be your main priority. You may also want to discuss a trust for minor children, which can take various forms. Many parents favour a discretionary trust, with their children and future grandchildren among the class of beneficiaries. Your solicitor will advise on the options here.

If the trust assets are not distributed by the time the youngest child reaches the age of twenty-one, a tax known as discretionary trust tax (DTT) arises. It is charged at 6 per cent of the value of the assets in the trust. For every year thereafter that the trust remains in existence, a further DTT charge of 1 per cent per annum arises. If the trust is fully wound up within five years of the initial 6 per cent charge arising, a refund of 50 per cent of the tax paid is made. Trustees may feel under pressure to distribute all of the assets from the trust by the time the youngest child reaches twenty-one to avoid triggering the charge. However, twenty-one is very young, and the trustees may decide that some of the assets should remain in trust if it appears to them that the children are not mature enough to be able to manage their inheritance outright at that stage.

Some parents direct that their estate is to be distributed between their children in equal shares absolutely on their death, but provide that it is to be managed on their behalf until they reach a specified age or until the children direct the trustees to hand the fund over to them. This can be attractive for tax purposes because any inheritance tax liability is paid immediately, and any later appreciation in value subsequently accrues directly to the children.

However, it carries with it the risk that if the children do not mature in the way the parent might expect, the decision to leave them substantial assets outright, with the trustees having no legal right to refuse to hand them over should they be requested to do so, might not be in the best long-term interests of the children.

Incapacitated children

If your child suffers from an incapacity of a permanent nature which prevents that child from managing his/her own affairs, a trust arrangement is likely to be essential to safeguard that child's best interests.

Adult children with vulnerabilities

You may have an adult child who does not suffer from an incapacity but who is vulnerable for some other reason. This may be an addiction, an acrimonious separation or divorce, or the child is simply hopeless at managing money. You may have to consider a trust arrangement in those circumstances. For example, the child could be given a life interest in specified property, meaning the child could receive the income generated by that property, or if it was a house or apartment the child could live there rent-free. However, the child would not be entitled to access the capital. The trustees could be given power to advance capital to the child in the future if they decided that this was appropriate. If the trustees were satisfied the child had matured, they could transfer the assets outright to the child and terminate the trust.

Adult child – no vulnerabilities

If your children are all mature adults with no disabilities or vulnerabilities, then you can make an outright gift or bequest to them, and there would be no reason to establish a trust. It is usually not tax efficient to implement trust arrangements for adult children.

Tax and other issues

Tax

You will want to consider structuring your will so that it is as tax efficient as possible.

Gifts or inheritances between spouses and civil partners are exempt from Irish gift and inheritance tax (known as capital acquisitions tax or CAT).

In all other cases, the recipient of a gift or inheritance (the beneficiary) is permitted to take a certain specified amount (the tax-free group threshold) free of CAT, depending on their relationship to the person providing the benefit (the disponer). Any excess over the tax-free group threshold is subject to CAT at 33 per cent unless a relief or exemption applies. The tax-free group thresholds are as follows:

Group	Relationship to Disponer	Exempt Thresholds 2021*
A	Son/Daughter/Stepchild or Son/Daughter of Civil Partner	€335,000
B	Brother/Sister/Niece/ Nephew/Grandchild	€32,500
C	Relationship other than Group A or B	€16,250

*All taxable benefits received from all donors on/after 5 December 1991 within this category must be taken into account in determining if the threshold has been reached.

In addition to the tax-free group threshold, a separate annual exemption of €3,000 per donor applies to all gifts (but not inheritances). Thus if you have four adult children, and you are in a financial position to do so, you can give gifts of €3,000 to each of them each year during your lifetime. These gifts are not taxable, and do not eat into the child's exempt threshold.

Other capital acquisitions tax exemptions and reliefs may apply, depending on the nature of the property you bequeath. For example, the dwelling house exemption can apply where a person has been living in a relevant dwelling house for a period of three years. Provided that certain conditions are satisfied, that dwelling house can be inherited free of CAT. One of the conditions is that the beneficiary cannot own or have an interest in another residential property at the time they inherit the house on which the exemption is claimed.

The dwelling house exemption is not limited to relatives. It could apply to a non-marital partner, for example.

Special categories of assets

If you have an interest in a business, particularly a complex one, you should consider how you would deal with the business in your will. What contingency plans are in place? Could your executors/trustees continue to carry on the business with the assistance of a management team? An orderly sale or wind-down of the business might be the best option, and you could give guidance on that. In other cases, it may be that a valued employee, associate or family member is available to take over the reins.

If you are a partner in a business or a shareholder in a company, your partner or co-shareholder may be one of your best friends and you may be tempted to name that person as executor or trustee of your will. You should hesitate before doing so, as potentially serious conflicts of interest could arise. For example, if it is decided that your interest in the business or company should be sold, he/she would be a potential purchaser, and cannot act on both sides of the transaction. It is preferable to have a written partnership agreement or shareholders' agreement dealing with the situation, if possible.

Foreign assets

If you own any foreign assets, you should check whether your Irish will can cover that asset, or whether you need to make a foreign will. You should also obtain advice on the tax and succession law rules in the country concerned.

Rights of cohabitants

If you have a partner with whom you cohabit, your partner may have a right to provision from your estate under the Civil Partnership and Certain Rights and Obligations of Cohabitants Act 2010. A cohabitant is one of two adults (whether of the same or opposite sex) who live together as a couple in an intimate and committed relationship. A cohabitant is only entitled to seek provision if that person is a qualified cohabitant, being a person who, immediately before the time that the relationship ended, whether through death or otherwise, had been living with the other adult for:

- two years or more, in the case where they are the parents of one or more dependent children; and

- five years or more in any other case.

A qualified cohabitant may seek provision, after the death of their partner, from the deceased's estate. The act does not confer an automatic entitlement to a specified share of a deceased's estate on the surviving cohabitant, who must initiate a court application to secure provision.

Cohabitants are subject to capital acquisitions tax on any benefits they receive as if they were strangers, except if it is obtained pursuant to a court order, in which case it will be exempt from CAT.

Cohabitants may enter into a cohabitants' agreement to provide for financial matters during their relationship or when their relationship ends, whether through death or otherwise. Cohabitants can opt out of the provisions of the act by executing a cohabitants' agreement stipulating their agreement on financial matters.

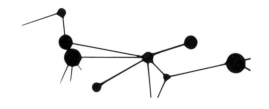

CHAPTER 10

The Role of the Irish Motor Neurone Disease Association and Other Supports Available

MAEVE LEAHY, TRACY HUTCHIN,
JOHANNA MCGRATH, FIDELMA RUTLEDGE

Introduction

The Irish Motor Neurone Disease Association (IMNDA) is the only support organisation in Ireland for people living with MND, their families, friends and carers. Since its foundation in 1985, the association has developed specialist, individualised services that reflect the needs of the Irish MND community. Our ethos is to ensure access to vital services for all people living with MND regardless of their demographic or means. Our main priority is to enable people with motor neurone disease to live as active, independent citizens within their community and to remain at home with their loved ones for as long as possible.

The IMNDA cannot slow the progression of MND or change the outcome, but we can help alleviate feelings of isolation and improve quality of life. If you or someone in your family has recently been diagnosed with motor neurone disease, it is likely that you are experiencing many confusing and confronting emotions. Good-quality information and support from people who understand MND is vital at this time. The MND community is extensive, committed and immensely supportive.

Our aim is:

- to encourage and promote the best methods of care, education, research and treatment for people with motor neurone disease throughout Ireland, contributing to worldwide efforts in research and development of treatments

- to establish and promote models of good practice in the delivery of specialised services to our patients, their families and caregivers, setting standards of excellence

- to communicate widely knowledge of motor neurone disease and related disorders in order to raise awareness in the wider community.

The IMNDA is here to help once you or someone you know has been diagnosed with MND. Our key services include:

- access to four MND nurses directly employed by the association
- access to specialised equipment on a loan basis
- access to a home care grant once recommended by the MND nurse and where a HSE home care package is ideally already in place
- counselling grant for the person with MND and one other member of their family
- freephone helpline 1800 403 403
- patient information booklet
- IMNDA community hub for online support
- funding and promotion of research into the causes and treatments of MND
- bereavement counselling grant.

So, how can we help you?

Whether you have been diagnosed with MND or you know someone who has, having access to our information services will make a huge difference to how you cope in the weeks and months ahead. MND is a life-changing illness and we are dedicated to making each change as smooth as possible for all those directly or indirectly living with it.

Providing information

The first step to living positively with MND is to gather information: what support is available; what to expect; how to cope, and so on. The more you know, the better you will be able to take control of what is happening to you and the care you receive.

It may be that you simply want someone to talk to. You might be concerned about a particular aspect of the disease and want to know more. You may be worried about the effect on your family. Or you might want to know as much as possible about MND, its causes, progress and treatment.

Whatever you need to know, we will do our best to help you:

- We operate a national freephone helpline Monday to Friday on 1800 403 403. This service offers accurate and up-to-date information on all aspects of MND.

- Once diagnosed, we provide all people living with MND with an information booklet. We also have more extensive literature that can be shared as required.

- Our website, www.imnda.ie, offers up-to-date news on developments alongside practical information on all aspects of living with MND.

No two people's experience of MND is the same. What affects one person may not affect another and so we try to meet each person's individual and unique needs. What affects one person in a family affects everyone in that family because receiving a diagnosis of motor neurone disease not only impacts on your life but on the lives of everyone around you. Adjustment takes time, and for many people living with MND, one of the most valuable sources of help is the MND nurse specialist. The nurse specialist has the experience and the knowledge to provide caring, practical support to you and your family.

IMNDA outreach nursing service

The four IMNDA nurses work alongside consultant neurologists throughout Ireland. As well as attending MND clinics, they travel around the country providing nursing support to people who have been diagnosed with MND. They provide support to their families and caregivers by means of home visits, a helpline, and online contact. All four nurses have a vast level of experience in the field of neurology and all have previously worked on the neurological ward in Beaumont hospital.

Being nurses that specialise in motor neurone disease means that not only do they play an active role in the lives of people living with MND, but they also share their expertise by way of educating local healthcare professionals to ensure that the highest level of patient care is being delivered at all times across the country.

The nursing service is active in its holistic approach to care, embracing physical, emotional, social and spiritual elements. It focuses on enhancement of quality of life for the person living with MND and their family and includes the management of distressing symptoms and provision of support and care throughout the journey of MND.

The MND nurses are central to the person with MND and their family. They are also a vital link to all of the services and healthcare professionals. They endeavour to coordinate a service that provides continuity of care for those living with MND and their caregivers in collaboration with community- and hospital-based healthcare professionals.

The IMNDA nurses have designated regional areas to ensure continuity of care and an equitable service throughout the country. They are there to:

- provide advice and support over the phone or via email

- visit you in your own home

- listen to your needs

- link you in with local services

- provide training and support to other healthcare professionals who are involved in your care.

Practical support

As MND progresses, everyday tasks may become more difficult. It could be something as simple as getting out of a chair, or you may have problems communicating should your speech be affected.

There is a wide range of equipment, technology and controls that can make a real difference to maintaining your independence and quality of life. Some of the key items are available through our equipment loan service.

These items are made readily available; however, it is important to note that you will need to be assessed, and the item must be requested by the appropriate healthcare professional from your multidisciplinary team (MDT), for example occupational therapist, speech and language therapist, assistive technology adviser or public health nurse.

If the IMNDA does not have the specialised item you require within its equipment stores and the item cannot be accessed through health or social services, the IMNDA may be able to fund the purchase of the required item.

Home care grant

The IMNDA can provide funding for care in the home. This funding is designed to act as a top-up to HSE-funded home care hours when the HSE hours are not sufficient to provide the level of care that is required for the client. This service can be requested through one of our MND nurses.

The IMNDA also provides funding for up to five nights of night nursing at the end-of-life stage of the disease. This is to be used as a top-up to the nights available through the Irish Hospice Foundation. Requests for this service must be received from the palliative care team in conjunction with the MND nurse.

Counselling grant

Diagnosis of an illness with a shortened life expectancy can lead to significant stress and anxiety, so appropriate referral to a qualified counselling service is essential.

The MND nurse will often suggest counselling for a person diagnosed with MND and the IMNDA funds six sessions, attended either alone or with another person. Every person diagnosed with MND will deal with it differently, and it is important to have the opportunity to talk about fears and concerns at the diagnosis of MND. For some it is not the fear of dying but the 'how will I die and when?' which affects most. For others it is the loss of the future that they thought they would have. The nurses try to navigate people through these various fears and emotions but they also rely on the expertise of experienced counsellors to help the individual and their family to cope with the news about the disease. Counsellors will advise on how to tell other family members, especially if there are young children in the family. For information about the IMNDA's counselling service, freephone 1800 403 403. The IMNDA also offers a grant for bereavement counselling for two family members or caregivers of an IMNDA client. Again, you can contact the office on freephone 1800 403 403.

Online MND support

Our IMNDA community hub is a safe and supportive online discussion site for people affected by motor neurone disease, their caregivers and families. Our community page allows you to post questions, share tips or advice, and interact with people with MND and their loved ones from around the country. Registration is free and your contact details are kept confidential. You can submit your own questions and use the answers provided by the community to help support you with MND. You will find our online community hub at http://community.imnda.ie/

What other help is available outside of the IMNDA supports?

Changes in life roles

As all the chapters in this book point out, everything changes for you and your family when you are diagnosed with MND. For example, younger members may be required to take on greater personal responsibility and household tasks, and adult members may be responsible for the majority of the care for their loved one. As advised in previous chapters, it is important to discuss how roles may change, and counselling can help with this.

Staying in work

A diagnosis of MND does not automatically mean that you will have to stop working. At the same time, it is better to be realistic about what you will or will not be able to continue doing. Physical jobs like building or decorating, for example, will become more difficult, more quickly, than desk-based jobs. Either way, it is important that you discuss your changed situation with your employer or human resources officer sooner rather than later. It may well be that you could work in a different area, reduce your hours, or modify your existing job.

Where to go for advice

The employment services officer at your local Intreo office can work with you and your employer so that you can continue working. Intreo offers the disabled worker and their employer a range of schemes and grants to cover workplace adaptation and employee retention.

For more information and to locate your local office, please go to www.welfare.ie

If you decide to stop work

If you feel you cannot continue working, carefully consider the options open to you. Can you take early retirement, or would you be financially better off if you took long-term sick leave for the maximum period possible?

Benefits and allowances

Disability allowance

Disability allowance is a weekly allowance paid to people with a disability who are between sixteen and sixty-six years of age. Disability allowance is a means-tested payment. To get the allowance, your total means must be below a certain amount, i.e. any cash income (both your own and your spouse), capital (savings, investments, shares, etc) and/or maintenance paid to you will be taken into consideration during the application for disability allowance.

If you qualify for disability allowance you may also get extra social welfare benefits with your payment and other supplementary welfare payments.

Illness (disability) benefit

You may get illness benefit if you cannot work because you are ill. Illness benefit was formerly known as disability benefit. The name of the benefit changed in 2006.

This benefit will vary depending on whether you are entitled to sick pay from work or not. Your employer can decide their own policy on sick pay and sick leave. You will need to check the policy around sick pay and sick leave in your workplace.

If you can receive sick pay from work, your employer will probably require you to sign over any illness benefit payment from the Department of Social Protection for as long as you receive sick pay from work. When your sick pay ends, your employer should stop getting your illness benefit.

Alternatively, if you are not entitled to sick pay from work, you may get illness benefit if you have enough pay-related social insurance (PRSI) contributions.

Invalidity pension

Invalidity pension is a weekly payment to people who cannot work because of a long-term illness or disability and who are covered by social insurance.

To be eligible, you must be in receipt of illness benefit for at least twelve months before you can claim invalidity pension. However, it may be possible to get invalidity pension after a shorter period if you are unlikely to be able to work for the rest of your life because of your illness or disability, which is fairly common for people with MND.

The invalidity pension is taxable and should be reported to your tax office as soon as your payment starts. You can contact the Revenue Commissioners at www.revenue.ie for more information. You may be entitled to a free travel pass and you may also get extra social welfare benefits.

Finally, some people do not feel that they are 'disabled' and think they are not entitled to make a claim. However, the term 'disabled' simply means that you have an illness that affects your ability to do everyday things. It is your right to claim these benefits if you meet the qualifying criteria.

For caregivers

Caring for someone with MND can be extremely physically and emotionally challenging. The IMNDA endeavours to support families and those with MND through this by providing counselling, funding for extra home care hours, practical advice, and encouragement. Despite how well many carers manage, the strain that many of them experience can be overwhelming and a break is imperative. MND nurses are very adept at noticing the signs of burnout in caregivers. Often our nurses will request respite in the hospice for a period to allow caregivers to 'recharge their batteries'.

As noted many times in this book, some people with MND may develop changes in thinking, reasoning and behaviour, and when this happens it can be very distressing for carers. The person with MND may appear to be selfish, to show poor empathy for their carers or their family, and be apathetic about what is happening around them. For families that experience this, the day services of the hospice can be their lifeline. This allows families time to understand these symptoms of MND, and be able to cope with them when the person returns home.

The day services of the hospice are extremely beneficial for those who opt to access them. Alternative therapies such as reflexology and art/music therapies are available, and the majority of people really enjoy them as well as having the opportunity to be with others who are dealing with their own battles. The hospice also gives people the opportunity to speak with a social worker who can assist with forward planning or other issues that may arise, such as access to a medical card.

Intimacy and MND

Physical intimacy in a relationship is an important touchstone for many couples, and it is not just about sex. It also encompasses activities that involve physical touch, such as holding hands, massage, kissing and cuddling. Following a diagnosis of MND, issues such as intimacy and sexuality are often not discussed, and this can have implications for many personal relationships. Many people feel embarrassed to ask their consultant or GP but they will ask the MND nurses about how it may affect them as the condition progresses. It is reassuring for people to know that MND has no direct link with fertility, libido, sexual arousal, or the ability to have an erection or an orgasm.

However, there are many factors that can affect a sexual relationship. The person with MND can experience fatigue associated with the condition, and their partner can be exhausted by all the daily routine tasks that were once shared. Caring for someone can be exhausting. Flexibility is very important, and finding a time when both people are rested can be an advantage.

Many people fear they may become breathless during sex, and this may be exacerbated by pressure on the chest or abdomen. It is possible to use non-invasive ventilation (NIV) during sex, and if the person would prefer not to, we advise them to keep it close at hand, to wear it afterwards.

It is also possible to have sexual relations when you have a PEG feeding tube. This is a common question we get asked when the decision is being made on whether to opt for the insertion of a PEG or RIG. It may be beneficial to tape the PEG to the skin prior to having sex and possibly wearing a fitted top to avoid it being dislodged.

If someone's mobility or movement is affected by MND, it may mean that their partner has to take a more physical role in lovemaking, such as a change of position, or activities such as massage. Even if someone has limited movement, their sense of touch is unaffected and so they can still enjoy the comfort and pleasure of touch.

The changes in someone's body as the disease progresses can be a source of huge distress and a person may feel less attractive and therefore feel their partner no longer finds them desirable. For a satisfactory sex life it is extremely important that these feelings are discussed. Telling your partner how you feel is important in maintaining intimacy. If a partner values the closeness and intimacy of kissing and cuddling, ensure the other partner knows, as they may value it more than ever now.

For further help and advice on care or intimacy, please consult your MND nurse.

Carer supports and benefits

Full-time caregivers may be entitled to support from the Department of Social Protection.

Carer's allowance

This is a means-tested benefit available to a caregiver providing full-time care to a qualifying person. The person being cared for must be incapacitated and require full-time care and attention and must be likely to require it for at least twelve months.

While receiving the allowance, a caregiver cannot be engaged in employment, self-employment, training or education courses outside the home for more than fifteen hours a week.

Assessment for the carer's allowance is based on any income you and your spouse/partner have, or property apart from your home, or an asset that could provide an income.

If you leave work to become a full-time caregiver and receive the carer's allowance, you will also be awarded PRSI credits.

Carer's benefit

This is a payment made to insured persons in Ireland who leave the workforce to care for a person(s) in need of full-time care and attention.

You are entitled to carer's benefit for up to a maximum of 104 weeks either over a continuous period or within a number of separate periods of time.

Income tax: home carer's tax credit

A tax credit may be available to married couples who are jointly assessed where one spouse is a home carer for someone who is over sixty-five or is permanently incapacitated. There are limits applicable to the level of income of the home carer.

The qualifying rules are complicated, so it is advisable to talk to the experts before applying. For more information and to obtain the IT 66 application form for home carer's tax credit, visit www.revenue.ie.

Medical card

The medical card is something we would recommend all clients with a diagnosis of MND to apply for as soon as possible for full access to health services. The medical card covers:

- free GP (family doctor) services

- prescribed drugs and medicines

- in-patient public hospital services, out-patient services and medical appliances

- some personal and social care services, for example public health nursing, social work services and other community care services.

For more information on benefits and entitlements relevant to you, go to www.citizensinformation.ie or www.welfare.ie

Getting around

Primary medical certificate

This certificate entitles its holder to a number of tax reliefs associated with buying or using an adapted vehicle for drivers and passengers with a disability. The tax reliefs include:

- remission or repayment of vehicle registration tax (VRT)

- repayment of value-added tax (VAT) on the purchase of a vehicle

- repayment of VAT on the cost of adapting a vehicle.

Disabled parking permit scheme

This scheme was born out of a basic necessity to maintain independence for people with limited mobility. A person with a disability requires access to a disabled parking bay because of its size (accessible parking bays are larger than the standard parking space) and their proximity to daily facilities. This gives vital access to work, shops, bank, social events, etc, that would otherwise severely restrict people with disabilities from participating in society.

The parking cards are issued by the Irish Wheelchair Association and the Disabled Drivers Association. Application forms are available from either organisation.

Nursing home support scheme

The Nursing Home Support Scheme, also known as the 'Fair Deal', provides financial support to people who need long-term nursing home care. The scheme is operated by the Health Service Executive (HSE) and replaces the nursing home subvention from 27 October 2009. Under this scheme you make a contribution towards the cost of your care and the state pays the balance.

The scheme covers approved private nursing homes, voluntary nursing homes and public nursing homes. You can find details of your local HSE Nursing Home Support Office at https://www2.hse.ie/services/fair-deal-scheme/contact-a-nursing-homes-support-office.html

Anyone who is ordinarily resident in the state and is assessed as needing long-term nursing home care can apply for the scheme. You can find details of the scheme at https://www2.hse.ie/services/fair-deal-scheme/about-the-fair-deal-scheme.html

Prescription costs

Under the Drugs Payment Scheme an individual or family, who reside in Ireland, are expected to pay a maximum of €114 (current rate) per month for approved prescribed drugs, medicines and certain appliances. Anything over this amount can be reclaimed using the Drugs Payment Scheme. Contact your local HSE health office for more information on this or visit www.hse.ie.

Medical card holders are entitled to approved prescribed drugs and medicines at a minimal cost (currently max €15 per person/family per month), so they are not eligible for this scheme. Applications for a medical card may be subject to a means test.

Housing and adapting your home

There are many practical things to consider when you have MND, such as the long-term suitability of your home or whether you should move, or renovate and stay where you are. There is often a great deal you can do to adapt your home to your changing needs, and the occupational therapist is the best person to speak to for advice. The *Housing Adaptation Grant for People with a Disability* can be used to help meet the cost of adapting a property for a disabled person, such as making your home wheelchair accessible, or allowing for the addition of a ground-floor bathroom or toilet or stair lift.

Your application will be assessed depending on medical need. There are three levels of need; ordinarily, a person with MND will fall into the highest priority level 1.

Unfortunately, the community HSE occupational therapist cannot complete your adaptation report. Your local authority may be able to arrange for an occupational therapist to visit your home, but, under the Housing Adaptation Grant for People with a Disability, you can employ an occupational therapist to carry out an assessment and recoup up to €200 as part of the total grant. For further information refer to the listings from the Association of Occupational Therapists of Ireland, www.aoti.ie.

If only minor work is required, you can apply for the *Mobility Aids Grant Scheme* instead. You must satisfy the means test to be eligible for the scheme and it is worth noting that you cannot receive both the Housing Adaptation Grant for People with a Disability and the Mobility Aids Grant Scheme.

For more information, visit www.citizensinformation.ie or contact your local authority.

Council tenants

Your local council may consider moving you to a more suitable property. Remember though that these are often in short supply and there is likely to be a waiting list. It is also worth talking to your social worker or Citizens Information centre for advice on available grants to help with the cost of fixtures and fittings you will need if you do move.

Financial advice

Anyone can find it difficult to manage their money even in ordinary circumstances. It can be particularly worrying if you unexpectedly find you cannot work and your income falls sharply.

Arrange a meeting with your bank or building society – they can only help if you talk to them.

If you have a mortgage, tell your mortgage lender about your changed circumstances and let them help you – again, they can only do so if you talk to them.

There are many charities, such as professional trade and benevolent funds or ex-service organisations, that will help with unexpected expenses – your local Citizens Information centre will have details.

Debt

Sometimes, getting into debt is unavoidable, but that doesn't make it any less stressful. Your local Citizens Information centre is a good place to go for advice, or you could contact one of the specialist advisory services such as MABS (Money Advice and Budgeting Service) Monday to Friday 9 a.m. – 8 p.m., www.mabs.ie.

Conclusion

There are myriad emotional tasks to be undertaken when you are told you have MND. However, the most important thing to know is that you and your family will be helped and supported every single step of the way. The evolving nature of the condition means that the expertise of all disciplines is required at various times throughout the condition. Everybody's needs vary, but the Irish Motor Neurone Disease Association

(IMNDA) is here to provide help regardless of when and how we are needed. We consistently support approximately 350 to 400 people with motor neurone disease at any one time. Our services are immediate and free of charge.

We do not just provide practical support and care. Our approach to MND is multifaceted. We also provide funding towards research on an annual basis; we fund scientific and medical research of the highest quality specific to MND. This research is conducted by Professor Orla Hardiman and her team in Trinity College.

The IMNDA is a small organisation achieving big things in the fight against MND. If you ever need support or advice, simply freephone 1800 403 403 or email services@imnda.ie.

We are here for all our MND community – now and always. 'Until there is a cure, there is care'.

GLOSSARY

Acetylcholine
A chemical in the brain and neuromuscular junction that acts as a neurotransmitter.

Adult stem cells
These cells are capable of replacing other cells which have died due to disease or injury.

Aggregation of cells
The clumping together of cells which may occur in response to abnormal changes to cellular structure.

Akinesia
Difficulty initiating purposeful movement, or the inability to do so.

Alleles
Forms of the same gene with small differences in their sequence of DNA bases. These small differences contribute to each person's unique physical features.

ALS
Amyotrophic lateral sclerosis (ALS) is the most common form of motor neurone disease (MND). It is a progressive neurological disorder which affects both the upper motor neurones in the brain and the lower motor neurones in the spinal cord, resulting in muscle weakness.

Amino acids
Amino acids are a group of small molecules which are the building blocks of proteins.

ANG (angiogenin) gene

The ANG gene provides instructions for making a protein called angiogenin. The physiological role of angiogenin is the formation of new blood vessels from pre-existing blood vessels through a process called angiogenesis.

Angiogenesis

A process which enables angiogenin to stimulate the growth and division of endothelial cells, which line the inside surface of blood vessels, to form new blood vessels. Angiogenesis is important for restoring blood flow after an injury.

Ataxia

Ataxia refers to a range of symptoms including difficulty with coordination, problems with targeted fine movements, and poor balance.

Atom

A particle of matter that uniquely defines a chemical element. An atom consists of a central nucleus that is usually surrounded by one or more electrons.

Atrophy

Atrophy refers to wasting and is most often used to describe volume loss in muscle and brain regions.

Autoimmune

Autoimmune processes refer to erroneous or overactive immune responses when the body's defensive cells and antibodies attack healthy cells and tissues.

Axon

Nerve fibres that conduct impulses from the neuronal cell body and connect to other cells, muscles or glands.

Beneficiary
A person who receives a benefit under a will or trust, or under the intestacy rules from the estate of a person who died without making a will.

Bilateral (B/l)
Refers to conditions and symptoms affecting both sides of the body, left and right.

Breath stacker
Breath stacking is a way to fill a person's lungs with more air than the person can usually take in when breathing naturally. Breath stacking helps people who have diminished lung capacity due to muscle weakness. Assisted breath stacking (e.g. using a lung volume recruitment bag with a one-way valve) is used for those with bulbar dysfunction or whose cough is ineffective with unassisted breath stacking.

Bulbar muscles
Muscles in the throat, voice box and neck that control speech, chewing and swallowing.

Bulbar symptoms
Symptoms involving the impairment of articulation and swallowing, which may be associated with excessive drooling.

Capital acquisitions tax
Tax imposed in Ireland on a person who receives a gift or inheritance.

Cell
A cell is the basic structural and functional unit of all organisms.

Central nervous system (CNS)
The brain and spinal cord.

Cerebrospinal fluid (CSF)
The protective fluid around the brain and the spinal cord, which can be analysed for a number of conditions.

Chromosome
Found in the nucleus of a cell, which contains the genes. Chromosomes come in pairs, and a normal human cell contains forty-six chromosomes.

Compound
A material made up of two or more elements.

Cough assist
The cough assist machine helps clear secretions by applying a positive pressure to fill the lungs, then quickly switching to a negative pressure to produce a high expiratory flow rate to stimulate a cough. This aids with secretion management and is often used in tandem with a suction machine to clear secretions following use from the oral cavity.

Dementia
Dementia is an umbrella term encompassing a multitude of conditions which are associated with the gradual deterioration of cognitive abilities and behavioural control.

Discretionary trust
A type of trust which gives the trustees power to decide how much of a trust fund will be distributed among the persons named as potential beneficiaries, and the manner in which it will be distributed.

DNA
A material found within the cell nucleus that is responsible for carrying genetic information. Each person has their own unique DNA.

DNA bank

A repository of DNA from people with MND and their unaffected carers/family. The bank provides a great resource for investigation into the genetic causes of MND.

Dysarthria

Difficulty with the articulation of words and sentences. Impaired speech that is characteristically slurred, slow and difficult to understand caused by paralysis, weakness, or inability to coordinate the muscles of the mouth.

Dysphagia

Difficulty swallowing solids and/or liquids.

Dyspnoea

Breathlessness.

Efferent nerve

A nerve that carries impulses from the central nervous system (CNS). An efferent nerve is the opposite of an afferent nerve that carries impulses towards the CNS.

Electrophysiology (neurological)

A collective term for the instrumental and quantitative assessment of nerve and muscle function, which is particularly informative in the diagnostic phase of MND.

Element

A simple substance which cannot be decomposed by chemical means.

EMG

Electromyography is an instrumental test used to assess the electrical activity of muscles. EMG is helpful in demonstrating lower motor neurone dysfunction in the diagnostic phase of ALS.

It can also detect subtle muscle twitching which is not visible to the naked eye.

Enzyme
A chemical that expedites various biochemical processes in the body.

Executor
A person appointed by will to administer the estate of a deceased person. Also known as a personal representative.

Fasciculations
Small, involuntary muscle contractions of individual muscle fibres which may be observed in the legs, arms, shoulders and tongue. It is very important to note that many people have fasciculations and these do not necessarily suggest ALS or MND.

Feeding tubes
A feeding tube is a medical device used to provide nutrition to patients who cannot obtain adequate daily calorie intake by swallowing. Various tubes exist depending on the mode of insertion, but irrespective of the type they all offer a safe way of administering nutrition. These tubes are not visible and are concealed under the clothing.

Frontotemporal dementia (FTD)
A disorder characterised by gradual cognitive and behavioural decline which may also be associated with language deficits, apathy and changes in personality.

Gene
A gene is the basic physical and functional unit of heredity, consisting of a segment of DNA arranged in a linear manner along a chromosome. Genes carry out instructions to make molecules called proteins. Every person has two copies of each gene, one of which is inherited from each parent.

Genetic
Inherited, having to do with information that is passed from parents to offspring through genes in sperm and egg cells.

Hemiplegia
One-sided weakness affecting the whole body, for example left arm and left leg weakness or right arm and leg weakness.

Humidification
Increasing the humidity of gases, such as in non-invasive ventilation, by the insertion of a water tank. This helps to keep the airways moist.

Hyperreflexia
Excessive response to muscle stretching when the reflexes are tested, such as the knee or ankle jerks.

Idiopathic
Of unknown cause. Any syndrome that is of uncertain or unknown origin may be termed idiopathic.

Inherited
A trait, condition or manifestation which is passed down from ancestors.

Kennedy's disease (spinal and bulbar muscular atrophy: SBMA)
A rare, genetic, progressive lower motor neurone disorder which typically affects men, and may have endocrine and cardiac manifestations in addition to muscle wasting, bulbar symptoms and tremors.

Lower motor neurones (LMN)
Neurones which originate from the brainstem or spinal cord and carry information to the muscles. They are under the command of the upper motor neurones (UMN).

Magnetic resonance imaging (MRI)
A medical imaging modality that provides high-resolution images of the body, including the brain, spinal cord and muscles. MRI does not use harmful X-rays and permits the careful evaluation of various brain and spinal cord structures.

Major gene
A gene that is necessary and sufficient by itself to cause a condition.

Mills disease
A rare motor neurone disease characterised by slowly progressive one-sided (left or right) muscle stiffness.

Nebuliser
A method of administering vaporised medications that can be inhaled.

Neurofibril
Long, thin, interlacing threads that run through the body of a neurone and extend into the axon and dendrites, giving the neurone support and shape.

Neurofilament
Neurofilaments are long, thin protein polymers found in the body and axon of neurones. They provide structural support for axons and impact on nerve conduction velocity.

Neuroimaging
A collection of modalities that facilitate the recording and interpretation of images from the brain and spinal cord, such as computed tomography (CT), magnetic resonance imaging (MRI) and magnetoencephalography (MEG).

Neurological
Having to do with the nerves or nervous system.

Neurone
The basic cellular unit of the nervous system. Most neurones are composed of a body, an axon and dendrites. The functions of neurones vary, but many of them contribute to the communication between the brain and the body; they are closely interconnected, forming complex neuronal networks.

Neurophysiology
The branch of clinical neuroscience concerned with recording and quantitative interpretation of electrical signals from the peripheral nerves, muscles, brain and spinal cord.

Neurotransmitter
A group of chemical substances that help communications between neurones as well as transmitting messages from neurones to muscles, glands and various other organs.

Neurotrophic factors
A family of proteins that induce the growth or survival of neurones.

NIPPV (non-invasive positive pressure ventilation)
An intervention that alleviates symptoms of breathlessness that can be used overnight or during the day as required. It works through a mask by providing extra air during inspiration. There are a multitude of machines available, most of them are quiet, portable and easy to use at home or during travel. Similar terms include NIV (non-invasive ventilation) or 'NIPPY'.

PEG (percutaneous endoscopic gastrostomy)
A thin concealed feeding tube which is inserted in the stomach during a small procedure called endoscopy, which is a camera inserted down the food pipe. It enables a person to receive food,

fluids and medicine directly when it is difficult or unsafe to use the normal route via the mouth.

Peptides
Compounds containing a sequence of 4 to 100 amino acid units, which are bound through at least one normal peptide link.

Peripheral nervous system (PNS)
The peripheral nervous system encompasses the nerves outside of the central nervous system (CNS). It connects the CNS to the organs, limbs and skin.

Primary lateral sclerosis (PLS)
A rare, relatively slowly progressive form of MND, which preferentially affects the upper motor neurones and manifests in lower limb stiffness, poor mobility and sometimes pseudobulbar affect.

Protein
Fundamental components of all living cells and include many substances, such as enzymes, hormones and antibodies, that are necessary for the proper functioning of an organism. They are compounds containing an amino acid sequence of more than 100 amino acids, at least two of which are different, bound mostly through normal peptide links.

Pseudobulbar affect (PBA)
Sudden, unprovoked or situation-inappropriate laughing or crying. An important symptom to discuss with the team, as a multitude of medications may alleviate these symptoms.

Ribonucleic acid (RNA)
A substance found in the cell nucleus which is responsible for regulating which genes are kept active. It serves as the intermediary between genes and the proteins that they code for.

RIG (radiologically inserted gastrostomy)
A thin concealed feeding tube which is inserted using radiological guidance.

SOD (superoxide dismutase)
An enzyme that inactivates excess free radicals, preventing them from damaging cell membranes. Mutations in SOD1 have been linked to familial forms of MND.

Synapse
The connection between two nerves or a nerve and other tissues (muscles, glands, etc) where a nerve impulse is passed from the end of the axon to another cell, such as a neurone, muscle, gland or other organ.

Testator
A person who has made a will.

Unilateral
Refers to conditions and symptoms exclusively affecting one side of the body, left or right.

Upper motor neurone (UMN)
Long, thin, specialised neurones located in the motor cortex in the brain. They regulate voluntary movement by sending messages down the spine, where they connect to the lower motor neurones (LMN), which ultimately connect to the muscles.

Viscosity
A measure of fluidity and thickness that can relate to a multitude of medical substances, blood, feeds, medications, secretions, etc.

OTHER RESOURCES

This information about services and supports, across public and voluntary sectors, has been compiled for readers, with particular emphasis on resources relevant to this book. However, the directory cannot be, nor does it claim to be, comprehensive, and further information about international or regional services may be obtained through websites.

In providing this list, no personal recommendation with regard to the services listed is made or implied by the author or by the publishers. While every effort has been made to ensure that the information given is accurate and up-to-date, no responsibility can be taken in the event of errors.

Additionally, it is always recommended that in any situation of concern people seek professional advice, and in relation to health or mental health that they consult their local general practitioner or health authority.

Academic Unit of Neurology at TCD:
https://www.tcd.ie/medicine/neurology
(Part of the School of Medicine, with close links to TCIN and the neurology units at St James's, Tallaght and Beaumont hospitals. Focuses on neurodegeneration, epilepsy, stroke medicine and neuropharmacology)

Age Action: **www.ageaction.ie**
(A national charity offering services and programmes to support older people and their families to live full and independent lives in their homes and communities)

All Ireland Institute of Hospice and Palliative Care (AIIHPC):
https://aiihpc.org
(Advances education, research and practice to improve the palliative care experience of people with life-limiting conditions and their families)

ALS Association: **www.als.org**
(An American association that provides information and assistance to people with amyotrophic lateral sclerosis)

American Psychological Association: **www.apa.org**
(Professional association for psychologists in the United States)

Australian Psychological Society: **www.psychology.org.au**
(Professional representative body for psychologists in Australia)

Aware: **www.aware.ie**
(Information and support on fear, anxiety and depression)

British Psychological Society: **www.bps.org.uk**
(A representative body for psychologists in the United Kingdom)

Canadian Psychological Association: **www.cpa.ca**
(The primary organisation representing psychologists throughout Canada)

Care Alliance Ireland: **https://www.carealliance.ie**
(National network of voluntary organisations supporting family carers)

Caring for Carers: **www.carers.thepalliativehub.com**
(Provides advice for carers and family caring for those with palliative care needs)

Central Remedial Clinic: **www.crc.ie**
(Provides a range of services and supports for people with disabilities, whether they are babies and toddlers, schoolchildren, teenagers or adults. Also supports for parents, carers and families)

Citizens Information: **www.citizensinformation.ie**
(Provides comprehensive information on public services and on the entitlements of citizens in Ireland)

Cognitive Behavioural Psychotherapy Ireland: **www.cbti.ie**
(Accreditation body for cognitive behavioural psychotherapy in
Ireland)

European Federation of Psychologists' Associations: **www.efpa.eu**
(Umbrella organisation for European psychological associations)

Family Carers Ireland: **www.familycarers.ie**
(Offers a range of services and support to family carers)

Family Therapy Association of Ireland:
www.familytherapyireland.com
(Information on therapy for individuals, couples and families)

Health Service Executive Carers Support:
www.hse.ie/eng/services/list/3/carerssupport (Specific
information on support for carers provided by the HSE)

Health Service Executive Services: **www.hse.ie/eng/services/list**
(Information on health and social services provided in Ireland by
the HSE)

International Alliance of ALS/MND Associations:
www.alsmndalliance.org
(Includes a directory of ALS/MND organisations worldwide)

Irish Association for Counselling and Psychotherapy: **www.iacp.ie**
(Professional association for counsellors and psychotherapists)

Irish Council for Psychotherapy: **www.psychotherapycouncil.ie**
(Information on psychotherapy services in Ireland)

Irish Hospice Foundation: **www.hospicefoundation.ie**
(A national charity dedicated to all matters relating to dying, death
and bereavement in Ireland. Provides essential services to help
people die well and grieve well)

Irish Motor Neurone Disease Association (IMNDA):
www.imnda.ie
(As this book conveys, the IMNDA provides care and support
to people with motor neurone disease, their families, friends and
caregivers)

Irish Wheelchair Association: **www.iwa.ie**
(Ireland's leading representative organisation and service provider
for people with physical disabilities)

Mental Health Ireland: **www.mentalhealthireland.ie**
(Advocacy and support for mental health)

Mindfulness and Relaxation Centre Beaumont Hospital:
www.beaumont.ie/marc
(Helping people cope with physical illness and ongoing medical
treatment)

MindYourSelf Series: **www.mindyourselfbooks.ie**
(Safe, researched, peer-reviewed self-care, health and well-being
book series)

MND Buddies: **https://www.mndbuddies.org**
(Online activity hub developed to give children aged 4 to 10
the chance to learn more about MND through games, stories,
activities and galleries)

MND Scotland Carers Hub:
https://www.mndscotland.org.uk/what-is-mnd/carers-hub
(Help and support for carers of people with MND as well as
funding vital research)

Motor Neurone Disease Association: **www.mndassociation.org**
(A UK charity which aims to improve access to care, research and
campaigns for those people living with or affected by MND in
England, Wales and Northern Ireland)

National Health Service: **www.nhs.uk**
(Publicly funded UK health service – supports include CBT and other forms of talking therapies for anxiety and stress)

Neurological Alliance of Ireland: **www.nai.ie**
(The national umbrella body representing over thirty not-for-profit organisations working with people with neurological conditions and their families)

Pieta House: **www.pieta.ie**
(Free support for those in suicidal distress)

Project MinE: **www.projectmine.com**
(An international project set up to understand the genetic basis of ALS, aiming to analyse the DNA of people with MND right across the world with the ultimate aim of finding a cure)

Psychological Society of Ireland: **www.psychologicalsociety.ie**
(Professional body for psychologists and psychology in the Republic of Ireland)

Research Motor Neurone: **www.rmn.ie**
(Promotes and facilitates research into the causes and treatments of motor neurone disease, and strives to increase awareness of the disease at both a national and international level)

Samaritans Ireland: **www.samaritans.org/samaritans-ireland**
(Confidential 24-hour telephone and online support for people who are depressed, suicidal or struggling to cope, or worried about someone else)

Smiling Mind: **https://www.smilingmind.com.au**
(Not-for-profit web and app-based meditation programme developed by psychologists and educators with links to a fully free mindfulness and meditation app)

St Francis Hospice: **www.sfh.ie**
(Provides a specialist palliative care service, including an in-patient unit, and home care and day care services, for the people of north Dublin city and county and surrounding counties)

The Palliative Hub: **https://thepalliativehub.com**
(Developed by the All Ireland Institute of Hospice and Palliative Care (AIIHPC) with a number of palliative and hospice care stakeholders, it acts as a gateway to information and resources about palliative care on the island of Ireland)

World Federation of Neurology Research Group on MND: **www.wfnals.org**
(Provides regular updates on scientific news relating to MND and ALS, and features a worldwide list of MND/ALS specialists and centres)

OTHER READING

Albom, M., *Tuesdays with Morrie: An old man, a young man and life's greatest lesson* (New York: Doubleday, 1997)

Cerutti, P., Solara, V. and Ferrario, S.R., 'Motorneurone Diseases: Impact on health professionals', *Giornale Italiano di Medicina del Lavoro ed Ergonomia*, vol. 38, no. 2, 2016, pp. 69–78

Christidi, F., Karavasilis, E., Rentzos, M., Kelekis, N., Evdokimidis, I. and Bede, P., 'Clinical and Radiological Markers of Extra-Motor Deficits in Amyotrophic Lateral Sclerosis', *Frontiers in Neurology*, vol. 9, 2018, art. 1005

Coote, T., *Live While You Can: A memoir of faith, hope and the power of acceptance* (Dublin: Hachette Books Ireland, 2019)

Finegan, E., Chipika, R.H., Shing, S.L.H., Hardiman, O. and Bede, P., 'Primary Lateral Sclerosis: A distinct entity or part of the ALS spectrum?', *Amyotrophic Lateral Sclerosis and Frontotemporal Degeneration*, vol. 20, nos. 3–4, 2019, pp. 133–45

Finegan, E., Chipika, R.H., Shing, S.L.H. et al., 'The Clinical and Radiological Profile of Primary Lateral Sclerosis: A population-based study', *Journal of Neurology*, vol. 266, no. 11, 2019, pp. 2718–33

Fitzmaurice, R., *I Found My Tribe* (London: Chatto & Windus, 2018)

Fitzmaurice, S., *It's Not Yet Dark* (Dublin: Hachette Books Ireland, 2015)

Hardiman, O., Doherty, C.P., Elamin, M. and Bede, P., *Neurodegenerative Disorders: A clinical guide*, 2nd edn (New York: Springer International Publishing, 2016)

Hennessy Anderson, N., Gluyas, C., Mathers, S., Hudson, P. and Ugalde, A., '"A monster that lives in our lives": Experiences of caregivers of people with motor neuron disease and identifying avenues for support', *BMJ Supportive and Palliative Care*, April 2016

Mancini, R.L. (ed.), *Motor Neurone Disease Research Progress* (New York: Nova Science Publishers, 2008)

McGovern, A., *Against the Odds: Living with motor neurone disease* (Dublin: Londubh Books, 2013)

O'Donnell-Ames, J. *The Stars that Shine* (Trenton, NJ: OpenDoor Publications, 2013)

O'Dwyer, M., *At the Coalface: A family guide to caring for older people in Ireland* (Dublin: Orpen Press, 2020)

O'Toole, S., 'Living and Dying with Motor Neurone Disease', unpublished PhD thesis, University College Dublin, 2011

Pinto-Grau, M., Donohoe, B., O'Connor, S., Murphy, L., Costello, E., Heverin, M., Vajda, A., Hardiman, O. and Pender, N., 'Patterns of Language Impairment in Early ALS', *Neurology: Clinical Practice*, 2020. DOI: https://doi.org/10.1212/CPJ.0000000000001006

Plummer, D., *Helping Children to Cope with Change, Stress and Anxiety (Activities Book)* (London: Jessica Kingsley Publishers, 2010)

Quinn, J., *Gratias: A little book of gratitude* (Dublin: Veritas, 2018)

Rabbitte, M., Bates, U. and Keane, M., 'Psychological and Psychotherapeutic Approaches for People with Motor Neuron Disease: A qualitative study', *Amyotrophic Lateral Sclerosis and Frontotemporal Degeneration*, vol. 16, nos. 5–6, 2015, pp. 303–8

Ray, R.A. and Street, A.F., 'Caregiver Bodywork: Family members' experiences of caring for a person with motor neurone disease', *Journal of Advanced Nursing*, vol. 56, no. 2, 2006, pp. 35–43

Rumi, *The Essential Rumi*, trans. by Coleman Barks (New York: Harper Collins, 1995)

Tolle, E., *The Power of Now* (London: Hodder & Stoughton, 2001)

Tolle E., *Oneness With All Life* (London: Penguin, 2020)

Tubridy, N., *Just One More Question: Stories from a life in neurology* (Dublin: Penguin Ireland, 2019)

Whyte, D., *Consolations: The solace, nourishment and underlying meaning of everyday words* (Langley, WA: Many Rivers Press, 2015)

INDEX